MULTIPLE SCLEROSIS

'Hope springs eternal from every page . . .
this is an excellent book and it offers hopeful
insight into this condition'

Nursing Times

'Remains the primary source of information
for patients'

Journal of the Society of Physiotherapy

'It represents the strongest challenge yet to
those who claim nothing can be done about
MS'

Natural Food Trader

By the same author:

EVENING PRIMROSE OIL

MULTIPLE SCLEROSIS

A Self-Help Guide to its Management

Judy Graham

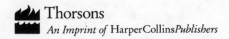
Thorsons
An Imprint of HarperCollins*Publishers*

Thorsons
An Imprint of HarperCollins*Publishers*
77–85 Fulham Palace Road,
Hammersmith, London W6 8JB

First published 1981
Second edition (enlarged) 1982
Third edition (revised) 1987
Fourth edition (completely revised and rewritten) 1992
This edition (revised) 1998
10   9   8   7   6

A catalogue record for this book
is available from the British Library

ISBN 0 7225 2777 2

Typeset by Harper Phototypesetters Limited
Northampton, England
Printed and bound in Great Britain by
Creative Print and Design (Wales), Ebbw Vale

Contents

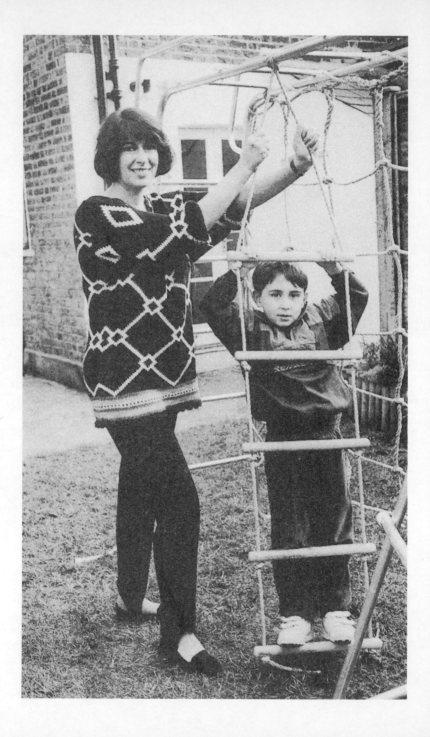

Dedication

For my darling son Pascal

'Le coeur a ses raisons que la raison ne connait point.'
                                                    (*Blaise Pascal*)

Acknowledgements

This book could not have been written without the help of a great many people. Very little in it is original material – I have simply gathered into one place all the various bits and pieces about the management of MS which have been written by other people elsewhere.

To credit all those people would fill several pages. But I would like to give a special thanks to Action and Research for Multiple Sclerosis, particularly everyone at the ARMS Research Unit at the Central Middlesex Hospital in London.

The inspiration for the book originally came from Joe Osborne of the Burton and South Derbyshire Independent Pool, to whom I give special thanks.

Many doctors have helped me with research material, books, and verbal advice. Some have written books of their own which are listed at the end. Personal thanks are due to Professor Michael Crawford; Professor Roy Swank; Professor EJ Field; Dr David F Horrobin; Dr Jurgen Mertin, Dr John Mansfield and Dr Patrick Kingsley. Two enlightened dentists also belong to this list – Jack Levenson and Vicky Lee.

Howard Kent, Lorraine de Souza, and Julia Segal did much of the original work in the chapters on yoga, physiotherapy, and mental attitude respectively. Muriel Tristant did the typing while I looked after my little son Pascal, or else looked after Pascal while I did the typing. This book would not have been finished without her willing help.

Lastly, my thanks to Pascal who put up with me fobbing him off while I worked, and to Michel, who has encouraged me in everything I do.

Foreword

This book by Judy Graham highlights the fact that anyone with multiple sclerosis can get better, or at the very least can prevent themselves from getting any worse.

Despite the knowledge that is available through the few doctors that have published their results, usually in a book for general reading, the vast majority of medical practitioners still see MS as an incurable condition and one which will eventually lead to life in a wheelchair for most sufferers, and ultimately death. As Judy Graham has done well with her own MS, but is not medically qualified herself, it suggests that her advice is better than that of most doctors.

I, for one, believe in her approach as the majority of the 1700 or so MS patients that I am seeing at present, who are also getting better, will attest to. Anyone who reads Judy Graham's latest book must surely be able to find in it something they can do to help themselves. The trick is to find out what is causing *your* MS.

When doctors do carefully controlled clinical trials, they try to apply the same 'treatments' to one group while a control group has no treatment at all. After an appropriate length of time, the outcome between the two groups is compared and statistics are applied to see if the 'treated' group did any better (or possibly worse) than the control group.

While this is the orthodox way of carrying out a clinical trial, and some would say it is essential to *prove* that any benefit wasn't just pure chance, it so often fails to demonstrate that the 'treated' group did get any better. This is because there wasn't enough overall improvement for the statistics to prove the point.

If 25 per cent definitely improved and the rest either got no better or continued to go downhill, the treatment would be considered a failure in the *whole* study. No-one would question whether those who improved had done so genuinely or not. The statisticians would say that their improvement was due to chance, and that the treatment was of no benefit to the 'treated' group as a whole.

The tragedy of this approach is that all MS sufferers are different. Their symptoms are different, their attacks and remissions are different, while some are the chronic progressive type and go downhill from the day of the first attack without any let-up. So how can groups be compared?

Far better to find out what is causing *your* MS and apply it to yourself, never mind the next person. In my experience an MS sufferer may have an allergy to milk, potatoes, wheat, citrus fruits, tea, or any number of other foods; a reaction to the amalgam filling in the teeth (but again some MS sufferers have had dentures since before their first attack); a gross deficiency of zinc, magnesium or B12, which they don't use properly even when given large supplemented doses; or any one of a number of anomalies. On the other hand only one or two of these may be important in your case.

I suggest you read this book through quickly first, just to get a feel of what it offers, then read it again picking out the parts you think could be relevant to you. Try to involve your general practitioner who will hopefully be pleased to do anything to try to help you, even if only to keep you quiet! Never give up.

My experience is that there always *is* a cause or causes for any ill-health, including MS. The problem is to find it. But you never will find it if you don't look. It's up to you to help yourself, and this book will help you.

Dr Patrick Kingsley, Leicestershire.
M.B., B.S., M.R.C.S., L.R.C.P., F.S.C.E., D.A., D.Obst., R.C.O.G.
British Society for Nutritional Medicine.
British Society for Allergy and Environmental Medicine.

Preface to the New Edition

I was diagnosed with MS eighteen years ago, and like any young person newly diagnosed I was fearful of the future.

How long would I be able to walk? Talk? See? Would I wake up one morning unable to move? How long would I be able to work? Would I ever become a mother? I can remember all these fears and anxieties as if they were yesterday.

At the age of 27, my MS symptoms were worrying enough to justify fears of getting worse. Sometimes I went numb along my left hand and arm and up to my face. At other times, both hands went very tingly and weak.

There were days when I couldn't feel my feet and could only tell what shoes I had on by looking. Sometimes I felt as though I were wearing leather boots up to my thighs while walking through a quagmire in the Arctic Circle. One sunny April I thought I had frostbite, my feet and legs were so frozen.

My walking was often horribly stiff, and I had to hold on to walls and furniture to keep my balance across a room. Some evenings I came home from work and simply flaked out on the sofa, not knowing why I felt so lifeless.

One nightmarish hot day I was faced by a steep flight of steps with no handrails, and I knew the only way I could possibly get down them would be on my bottom or leaning on someone's arm. It truly felt as if I was on the slippery slope, the only way being down.

At 27, I felt more like 87, hobbling about like an old lady and despairing at my stolen youth.

As I write this now, the picture is very different.

I don't hobble, I'm not numb anywhere, I can feel my hands

and feet, they're never cold, I don't need to hold on to walls and furniture, and I don't flake out.

My present job as editor of a daily TV programme and manager of a department in a television company is high-powered, with 10-hour days and constant pressure.

At home, there is little time to take it easy, what with my very energetic seven-year-old son Pascal, a house to run, meals to cook and so on.

To the casual observer, I lead a life normal enough to career women in their mid-40s, juggling career, child, partner and home. It's only under closer scrutiny that someone would notice that it's my nanny – and not me – who is playing with Pascal, because I cannot run, and someone else who is cleaning my house because I don't have the energy to do that as well.

The reason I emphasize how normal my life is now is to give hope to young people who have recently been told they've got MS and who don't want their future blighted by the illness.

If nothing else, I am living proof that you don't have to get worse once you have MS. It is possible to stabilize, and even to improve.

So what have I done to control MS? This book describes in detail all of the things that one could possibly do to help control the disease. Some of them I have done, some of them I used to do or else do spasmodically, some of them I have not needed to do, and some of them I still do today.

Of course, sceptical doctors will dismiss this, saying that MS is an unpredictable disease with ups and downs, and that some people have a benign course, or that symptoms can disappear just like that anyway, and that there is no treatment of proven benefit in MS.

Within myself, I feel certain that the various therapies I have been doing have contributed to my improvement. It is not just luck. The very fact that you are reading this book at all suggests that you are at least open to the idea that there might be things which can help you if you have MS. My hope is that, once having read the book, you'll be convinced enough to do some of these things. After all sceptical doctors have virtually nothing to offer. This self-help programme has many things to offer.

I began researching self-help therapies for MS almost as soon as I was diagnosed. This coincided with the formation of the Multiple Sclerosis Action Group (later to become ARMS) which had its first meeting in my London flat.

One of the first research projects funded by the MS Action Group was work by Professor EJ Field into evening primrose oil and MS. I started taking evening primrose oil capsules in 1974 and have been taking them every day since then, plus a variety of vitamin and mineral supplements (for the full list see chapter 8.)

The MS Action Group also backed research by a specialist in brain lipids, (now) Professor Michael Crawford. He worked out a diet which is high in essential fatty acids and nutrients, and low in saturated fat. This was the basis of the present ARMS Essential Fatty Acids Diet. I switched to this diet, and then had my blood monitored for changes. And, sure enough, the essential fatty acid profile of my blood gradually changed from abnormal to normal.

Shifting from a high saturated fat to a high polyunsaturated fat diet is probably the most important component of the self-help programme.

A few years ago, I consulted a doctor trained in allergy and Environmental Medicine, Dr Patrick Kingsley, who has had much success with MS patients. He advised me to give up tea, coffee, sugar, milk and milk products, and yeast. Even though I had not felt too bad while eating all of these things, there was a dramatic effect almost overnight when I gave all of them up. It was like a sort of fog lifting, and had a dramatic effect on banishing fatigue. He also advised weekly injections of Vitamin B12.

The more I learn about MS, the more I am convinced that food sensitivity and other environmental allergies[1] do play a part. Discovering exactly which foods or environmental agents you may be sensitive to may be a matter of trial or error. But it will be worth it.

As for exercise, I have to admit that I have fluctuated in my adherence to an exercise regime, even though I am convinced that sticking to a regular exercise programme is the right thing to do.

During those times when I have done regular exercise or practised yoga, I have noticed the benefits in terms of fitness, suppleness and increased stamina. During my lazy periods, I have noticed how stiff I am by comparison. There seems no doubt that gentle exercise, stopping before you get tired, really does help.

About seven years ago I had a course of hyperbaric oxygen. This did make me feel full of energy. However, as I had no bad symptoms at the time, it was difficult to measure improvements.

1. For a definition of 'allergy' in this context please see page 111.

For several years, I was treated by an acupuncturist, who is also an osteopath and homoeopath. I have also had deep massage treatment from time to time. All these 'alternative' therapies have helped.

This book covers an all-embracing approach to MS. People sometimes ask me in exasperated tones how I know which thing is doing any good when there are so many of them. But the idea is not to conduct some kind of scientific experiment as if one were testing a drug. I do not agree with the mechanistic approach to medicine anyway. Quite possibly, the self-help therapies in this book work together as a total lifestyle.

Once you start researching multiple sclerosis, you very quickly discover that many people who are involved with MS back different horses when it comes to treatment or management of the disease. Some people, for example, get evangelical about hyperbaric oxygen treatment, others about allergies, others about diet. Once people become religious about their own chosen therapy, they think they have seen The Way and The Light, and that everyone else is wrong, misguided, mad, mistaken, and barking up the wrong tree.

It has been my privilege over the years to be allowed to see at first hand each of these groups, thus becoming aware why certain people feel very 'pro' about their way of treating MS and equally 'anti' about other ways. Taking a broad overview, I have been truly eclectic in my approach.

As a journalist, I have been careful not to align myself too closely with any one therapy. Although I am a member of both ARMS and the MS Society, I do not necessarily share their policy viewpoints (or indeed they mine).

All opinions and conclusions in this book are my own. I have no financial, business, or other interest in any of the companies listed in this book. I mention this because some of my critics have hinted that anyone who espouses the attitudes described in this book must be in it for the money. This is untrue.

There is no suggestion that anything in this book constitutes a 'cure', though it could well be called 'healing'. My own view is that, because MS seems to be such a multi-factorial disease, one 'cure' – in the way you might take an antibiotic to cure an infection – is just not plausible for a disease of this nature.

Rather, you have to find whatever it may be that may have contributed to your disease in the first place – and the first place could go back several years – and replace those things which were doing you harm with things which will do you good. This may include removing stress and changing mental attitudes as much as changing diet.

I certainly wish that a book like this had existed when I knew nothing of MS back in 1974. My wish is that this book will satisfy a sorely felt need, particularly that of newly-diagnosed people all over the world. If doctors are failing to answer this need, then we must do it ourselves.

Introduction

Many people with MS are more disabled than they need to be. Many people with MS are getting worse, when right now they could be getting better.

It is truly a scandal that doctors often wait for a patient with MS to become visibly disabled before making a diagnosis (if they make one at all). It is a scandal because the earlier a patient is diagnosed, and the earlier the patient starts any treatment, the more successful it is likely to be. Most MS patients are being denied this opportunity.

Doctors have some stock reactions to finding out that a patient has MS. Some still don't tell the patient that he or she has MS, fobbing them off with some explanation for the symptoms. Others diagnose MS on the patient's notes, but don't tell the patient. They justify this by saying that there is no point in telling the patient because nothing can be done anyway, and a diagnosis of MS could send the patient into a terrible depression or even lead to suicide. Another stock response is to tell the patient that he or she has MS but then say 'Go away and forget about it,' or else 'I'm sorry, there is nothing we can do for you.'

All of these responses are based on the doctor's belief that MS is a chronic disease for which there is no known cause, cure or treatment. The result of this belief is that many thousands of people with MS are allowed to get worse. One could even dare suggest that certain procedures or treatments done in the name of medicine actually accelerate the deterioration of MS sufferers.

Surely the aim of medicine should be to treat an illness at the earliest opportunity, before it has taken hold, rather than wait for it to develop into a chronic illness? By and large, however, waiting is what is happening now, the world over, with multiple sclerosis.

The record of orthodox medicine in regard to MS has been poor. Other ways now need to be found. For too long, doctors have gone along with the received wisdom about MS – that there is no known cause, cure or treatment. This received wisdom must now be challenged on several scores. This book takes up that challenge.

My view in this book is that there are probably several causes of MS. There may be clues in the medical history, diet, lifestyle, stresses and attitudes of each person with MS, if only we look for them. Many factors may be involved in causing MS.

If that is so, it is most unlikely that there can be a single cure for such a multi-factorial disease. I believe that the concept of 'cure' is not helpful, as it is based on the idea that a drug can be a magic bullet, in the way that an antibiotic can cure an infection. I cannot see how this can apply to multiple sclerosis.

Instead, one can think of recovering one's health and well-being, being healed, which I believe *is* possible. I believe that there are several treatments that can bring about this increase in health and well-being. I doubt that any one drug treatment is ever likely to bring this about.

The treatments, or management programmes described in this book involve every aspect and layer of life. These treatments may not have been rigorously tested by scientific method, but we now have enough studies and enough anecdotal evidence to suggest strongly that the progression of MS can be slowed down, halted, or even reversed.

The kinds of therapies listed in this book do not lend themselves to the rigorous double-blind controlled trials beloved of scientists. They are not drugs and cannot be tested as if they were.

Moreover, doctors are always saying that no two cases of MS are alike. If that is so, how can they possibly bunch together 200 or 300 MS cases for a trial, and how can they possibly match them against controls? This stumbling block has always baffled me when doctors start waving their 'there is no scientific evidence' finger at me. And, quite apart from anything else, many people consider it unethical to deprive the control group of a therapy they are convinced is of benefit.

It is true that nothing in this book can be described as scientific proof, although certain studies, as you will see, do deserve to be taken very seriously. Cast-iron scientific proof is what doctors are waiting for. While they wait, however, thousands of people with

MS are getting worse, many of them perhaps needlessly.

If anecdotal evidence were not treated with such unjustifiable derision and if the medical profession would take a more flexible approach and see each patient as an individual, see healing as an art *and* a science, and stop dividing the body into pigeonholes, thousands of patients would benefit.

It is nothing short of a scandal that doctors do so little to help MS patients. When you go to see your doctor as an MS patient, the doctor should be able to say to you 'Yes, there are many things we can do to help you. There is a special diet that helps; there are vitamins, minerals and other supplements I can prescribe that might help; I can refer you to a physiotherapist at the local hospital; you can go to a local gym; if you have any bladder problems I can refer you to a urologist who can treat them; I can have your blood tested for allergies; I can give you a B12 injection regularly; and we run a yoga class on Fridays.'

Unfortunately, I doubt that there is a single doctor who says this.

As things stand at the moment, the more usual picture is for patients to go to their doctor and mention that they are on a special diet or taking supplements. Although some of these supplements are prescribable, they are not easy to get, so doctors tend to just let such patients get on with it, in a *laissez-faire* sort of way.

Of course, doctors may prescribe drugs. Corticosteroids such as prednisolone work as immunosuppressants. When there is a flare-up, corticosteroids work by dampening it down. Drugs such as this are effective in the short term, but I do not believe that they are the answer in the long term. Drugs like this do have side-effects, which are cumulative. These side-effects include 'moon face', superfluous hair, and candidiasis. Immunosuppressive drugs also weaken the immune system.

The aim of everything in this book is to do the exact opposite – to strengthen the immune system without resorting to drugs.

This book is a self-help guide. How much better our health system would be if patients with a chronic disease like MS did not have to rely on *self*-help to *get* help. Doctors tend to think that MS is an incurable and chronic disease and that there is nothing they can do. I believe that when you put all the facts together – as I have done in this book – you have to reach the more hopeful conclusion that there are things that can help.

After reading this book, you may decide to take a bolder approach with your doctor and ask to be referred to specialists who can help you. It is iniquitous, for example, that so few patients are referred to a physiotherapist *at a time when they can still be helped*.

The time has come to stir up doctors and convince them that they have an important part to play in the management of multiple sclerosis.

Self-help alone is not enough, but it does have certain virtues. It means that you decide to do something to help yourself, rather than have others do things for you. That decision to help yourself will make you feel much more positive.

Those who have been told they have MS should also be told that many, many people with MS have managed to stay well by following certain guidelines. Surely this is better than a sentence of slowly getting worse and worse, with nothing that can be done.

It cannot be guaranteed that doing the things in this book will stop you from getting worse, but the suggestions are worth a try. At the very least, this book suggests a healthy way of life.

For many – if not all – something *can* be done. This book tells you what, and how.

1

What Exactly is MS?

SIGNS AND SYMPTOMS OF MS

Whatever the causes and mechanisms involved in MS may be, the main effects of MS are on the central nervous system, which means the brain and the spinal cord. This is why MS is classified as a neurological disease and is the specialty of neurologists.

Symptoms can include any or all of the following: tingling, or pins and needles, anywhere in the body; difficulty in walking; dragging either foot; loss of co-ordination; loss of sensation or distorted sensation anywhere in the body; numbness in the hands, feet, limbs or other parts of the body; feeling like you are made of cotton wool, rubber or jelly; clumsiness; double or blurred vision or temporary blindness in an eye; slurred speech; an urgency to urinate or an inability to pass urine; loss of balance; unnatural fatigue; a feeling of tight bands around the trunk or lower limbs which can be itchy; sometimes pain; vertigo; tremors in the hands and arms; spasticity of the muscles or else muscles like jelly; a feeling of extreme cold like frostbite in the extremities; feeling like a wet rag in humid weather.

The Course of MS

Usually, the only type of MS mentioned is the relapsing-remitting type, where someone has an attack, followed by a remission, when the person goes back to the way he or she was before the last attack, or slightly worse than before. Scientists have been trying to find out just what it is which switches people into a remission. Many have felt that if only they could solve the mystery of remission they could treat MS.

The relapsing-remitting type is by no means the only course of MS. The other common type is described by scientists as 'chronic progressive'. In these cases, there are no clear-cut 'attacks' and the person just gets progressively worse.

In some rare cases, it is possible to get a galloping form of MS, where the person degenerates rapidly and dies within a few years. But it is also possible to have one attack of MS, and then to have nothing happen to you ever again, and live to a ripe old age.

Doctors sometimes say that the first five years of MS are a predictor of the future. Those who have hardly got worse in that time are said to have a 'benign' course.

The aim of this book is to do something about the disease early on so that one is not faced with the horrible prospect of getting worse and worse, at whatever speed.

The Cause, or Causes of MS

What causes MS, and what is going on in MS, are a complex puzzle. One scientist has described MS as 'baroque in its complexity'.

As the years roll by, the puzzle just seems to grow more complex – immunoglobulins, abnormal IgG ratios, monoclonal antibodies, histocompatibility antigens . . . How all these pieces fit together has not yet been solved by scientists. However, this book is not the place to try and unravel the complex mechanisms that are going on in the disease. What is important to know is that there are some broadly undisputed facts about what is going on in MS which make this self-help programme relevant. I will describe these in a moment.

However, it is useful to know the orthodox theories about MS as they now stand.

The prevailing wisdom among orthodox doctors in the field of MS is that MS is a multi-factorial disease. They believe that a virus, or viruses, may be the infecting agent, and there is some evidence that people with MS have an intrinsic inability to cope with such viruses. The immune system plays a complicated part in all this, perhaps causing the scattered damage to the nervous system.

Epidemiological studies (studies done on different populations in different parts of the world) suggest that there may be some environmental agent at work in MS. Other studies point to some genetic component.

Large amounts of money are being spent on medical research targeted at these areas. The aim is to find the cause or causes of MS first, so that a treatment or treatments can then be found, and finally a cure, or a prevention, or both.

While all these global theories may well turn out to be true, a more holistic approach would be to look for more personal reasons for your disease, or dis-ease.

There may be stress factors in your life which triggered the first symptoms. There may also be environmental factors which affect you in an individual way. You are the only person who can discover the more personal causes of why you have MS. A voyage of self-discovery may help answer deep questions about 'Why me?' and, once revealed, help you on your journey to health.

The global theories about MS may take years to come to fruition. I believe we have enough knowledge *now* about what is happening in MS to start self-help treatment without losing precious time.

What is happening in MS?

There are some medical facts about MS which have been pieced together and which are for the most part undisputed, and helpful to know.

Myelin and Demyelination

The central thing that is happening in MS is that myelin is breaking down. Everyone agrees about that. But what scientists don't agree on is *why* the myelin breaks down and whether this breakdown of myelin is the primary event in MS, or whether it follows on from something else happening.

MS is a disease which affects the central nervous system. The central nervous system is the brain and the spinal cord. In the white matter of the central nervous system (CNS) each nerve fibre (called an axon) is surrounded by a layer of insulation, called myelin. Nerve signals cannot travel normally without this insulating sheath, and without myelin there may be faulty connections between adjacent nerve fibres.

Think of these myelin-covered nerve fibres as if they were an electrical cable containing many wires. In a cable, it is very important that the wires should not make contact with each other. To stop this from happening, each wire is covered by some insulating material – usually rubber or plastic. The insulation makes sure the electricity in the wire goes to its destination without short-circuiting.

In multiple sclerosis, the myelin in the central nervous system suffers patches of demyelination. The damage to the brain and spinal cord occurs in many widely scattered areas. That is why it is called 'multiple' – there are many patches of damage. The damaged area becomes filled with hard material, or scars. 'Sclerosis' means scars. Multiple sclerosis means many scars. How your MS affects you may depend on where in the brain and spinal cord the scarring, or plaques, are.

It is the white matter of the brain and spinal cord which is damaged in MS, rather than the grey matter. The white matter actually looks white to the naked eye. It consists of fibres which carry messages from the sense organs – like the skin, eyes and ears – up to the higher parts of the brain. The white matter also sends messages from the brain down to the muscles.

The white matter also links up various parts of the brain. It is the sort of 'wiring' of the brain. This explains why your ability to feel, move, and co-ordinate is affected in MS.

Even though demyelination in MS still leaves many questions unanswered, more is known now about myelin and its breakdown than even five years ago. Seventy-eight per cent of myelin is made up of lipids, which are complex fats. Myelin also contains proteins. (You will see later in the book that the best nutrition for MS is very rich in the kind of structural fats which go to make up myelin.)

MS *only* involves demyelination of the central nervous system. The nerve fibres in the peripheral nervous system do not get affected in MS. The myelin in both systems is similar in its lipid composition. But the two types of myelin are quite different in their protein composition. The other big difference is that in the central nervous system there are glial (special connective tissue) cells called oligodendrocytes which are responsible for producing myelin sheath, whereas in the peripheral nervous system there are other types of cells which do this, called the Schwann cells.

Myelin Breakdown Under the Microscope

Scientists are now able to see clearly for themselves what is going on when myelin breaks down.

They have identified in particular something called a *macrophage*. In normal circumstances, macrophages are goodies. They are mobile white cells present in the blood which infiltrate into damaged tissue. They aid other troops in the immune system to remove debris and bacteria by scavenging them, or gulping them up.

It now seems that myelin breakdown only seems to occur in the presence of infiltrating macrophages. Under the microscope, these macrophages can be seen actually gobbling up the myelin. MS is called an auto-immune disease because components of the immune system turn against the body instead of defending it. These rogue macrophages are part of the auto-immune process in multiple sclerosis. Why the macrophages decide to turn on myelin is still a puzzle. Other bits of the immune system, such as the lymphocytes, are thought to behave in a hostile way too.

Then there are the *astrocytes*. Astrocytes are the cells that form the scar after the myelin is destroyed. But they are turning out to be baddies too. They produce enzymes which are a bit similar to macrophages in that they are garbage collectors – they clear away dead and waste products. It now seems that these enzymes may play an important role in damaging myelin in an area of inflammation. This inflammation itself is a key part of an acute attack in MS. Moreover, the myelin contains an enzyme system of its own which can digest myelin proteins and contribute to breakdown.

The switch, or trigger, that switches these processes on is still open to debate. In any case, some scientists hold the view that it is futile to look for any trigger, as the process of demyelination is a purely degenerative one. This means that the myelin itself degenerates without any trigger because it was never properly built in the first place. The building blocks for laying down strong myelin were faulty and it did not have the strength to last a lifetime, as it normally should. The building blocks which lay down strong and healthy myelin are largely made of structural fats.

Myelin Can Regenerate

Whatever the reason or reasons for myelin breaking down, the heartening thing to know is that myelin can regenerate. Not long ago, it was thought that myelin could not regenerate, but now this seems to be mistaken. Although myelin is a relatively stable structure, individual components do turn over, with old components being broken down and replaced with newly-formed components.

This means that some of the damage sustained by the nervous system is in principle capable of recovery. MS plaques may not be fixed sites of permanent damage, but areas in which damaged tissues are attempting self-repair. The trick is to know exactly what conditions aid that recovery. Some, or a combination, of the therapies featured in this book may be providing these conditions which aid myelin regeneration.

For a long time, researchers have been saying that if only they could find out what made myelin regenerate, they could solve MS.

The Myelin Project

Since 1990 the Myelin Project has been collaborating in international research aimed at repairing myelin.

For further information:

The British Trust for the Myelin Project
4 Cammo Walk
Edinburgh EH4 8AN
Tel: 0131-339 1316

Other Ideas About the Mechanisms Involved in MS

An Inborn Mishandling of Essential Fatty Acids

As long ago as the 1960s, a British scientist called RHS Thompson came up with the brilliant hypothesis that MS may develop against a background of inborn mishandling of certain essential fatty acids. This has been called 'Thompson's anomaly'. The significance of this anomaly is that the 'soil' is prepared for the development of MS. Because of this mishandling of essential fatty acids, *all* the cells in the body are abnormal, and myelin is built in such a weak way that it is prone to degeneration, falling to pieces rather like a badly-built wall.

An Inability to Handle Saturated Fats

Professor Roy Swank, champion of the low-fat diet, believes that the bunching together of platelets – caused by a diet high in saturated fats – stretches the blood vessel walls. This leads to a loss of integrity of the vessel walls, and in time toxic materials are able to seep through the blood into the brain. Professor Michael Crawford, who is behind the ARMS low-fat diet, goes along similar lines.

So according to Swank, MS is primarily due to an unstable blood emulsion from excess intake of fat in susceptible people. This susceptibility might be a defect in the red cell membrane, or a plasma abnormality.

Breakdown of the Blood–Brain Barrier

There is now widespread agreement that MS plaques are associated with, and form around, very small veins – or venules – within the central nervous system. These 'perivenular' plaques seem to happen when the blood–brain barrier is breached.

Blood is not supposed to cross over into the brain. There are potentially harmful substances carried in the blood, which must be kept away from the central nervous system. If blood does get across the barrier, it is toxic to nerve tissue.

The walls of the blood vessels which supply the nervous system – called the endothelium – have a special structure and way of functioning which makes it a barrier against harmful substances.

But at the same time this membrane allows necessary nutrients and gases to pass through it.

It seems that when there is a breach in the blood–brain barrier, it is followed by a local swelling, the breakdown of myelin, an inflammatory macrophage response, and the formation of a central hardened zone of fibrous material.

Several researchers working in the field of MS have come to the conclusion that the primary event which is happening in MS is the breach of the blood–brain barrier. So this is the first thing which should be stopped. The other events which are known to be happening in MS, such as the breakdown of myelin or rogue macrophages on the rampage, only seem to be happening *after* the blood–brain barrier has been broken.

Dr Philip James, champion of hyperbaric oxygen treatment for MS, believes that fat embolism is responsible for the breach in the blood–brain barrier. This is explained more fully in the chapter on HBO, chapter 13.

Broadly speaking, several theories agree that *fat* is to blame for damaging the vessel walls. But there is also some evidence that other things can weaken the blood–brain barrier intermittently, and so allow stuff from the blood to leak through to the brain. These things include:

*   Stressful events
*   Fatigue
*   Fever
*   Emotional upsets
*   Heat
*   Injury.

All events such as these provoke a physiological coping response which includes the release of adrenalin. This brings about arousal and mobilization of bodily resources. Part of this involves an increase in blood supply to the CNS. But there is also increased blood–brain barrier permeability. Anyone who has had attacks of MS knows that the above list of 'stressors' often precipitate attacks.

Mercury, a nerve poison, can also get across the blood–brain barrier (see chapter 11).

The aim of some of the therapies featured in this book is to prevent the primary reason for the blood–brain barrier being breached.

Is There an Abnormality in the Blood of MS People?

One hypothesis is that people with MS have abnormally-shaped red blood cells, which in turn makes the blood flow abnormal. This in turn leads to a complex sequence of events in which the blood–brain barrier is breached, demyelination takes place and plaques form.

According to Dr LO Simpson of the Otago Medical School in Dunedin, New Zealand, this abnormality in red blood cells and blood flow is the *primary* dysfunction in MS, which *leads* to neurological and other problems.

Dr Simpson believes that typical MS symptoms such as blurred vision after exertion, cold hands and feet, and fatigue, can best be explained by poor peripheral blood flow in the capillaries.

Other researchers have also found abnormalities in the blood of MS patients.

Under the microscope, Dr Simpson found that the red blood cells of MS patients were misshapen. Healthy red blood cells are supposed to be disc-shaped, but the MS red blood cells he had under the microscope can best be described as wonky.

Dr Simpson does not put forward a hypothesis as to why people with MS have abnormally-shaped red blood cells. However, he feels that in the light of his findings, MS research should take a new direction. It has been concentrating most of its efforts on neurology and immunology. Dr Simpson feels that MS researchers should now look first and foremost at haematology and focus research on treatments which would normalize red blood cells.

He and other researchers have been doing work on the effect of polyunsaturated fatty acids (PUFAs) on red blood cells. It seems PUFAs may be able to normalize these cells.

The question which has to be answered is: if PUFAs do normalize red blood cells, does this halt the whole MS disease process?

My own view is that it is well worth taking a diet rich in PUFAs now, without waiting for the medical researchers to come up with definitive answers, which could take a very long time indeed.

Research carried out in 1991 by Dr Rosie Jones and others at Bristol Royal Infirmary, using the electrophoretic mobility test, shows that there is an abnormal fatty acid content in the cell membranes of people with MS. They are particularly low in linoleic acid and arachidonic acid. Whether these low levels are part of the *cause* of MS has yet to be established, says Dr Jones.

WHY DIAGNOSING MS IS SO IMPORTANT

MS is notoriously difficult to diagnose clinically, partly because MS symptoms can also be the symptoms of other diseases. However, there are new techniques for diagnosing MS.

It is important to diagnose MS for the following reasons:

* To exclude the possibility of other illnesses which could be effectively treated.
* To start a management programme before the disease progresses.
* To be referred to specialized therapists, e.g. physiotherapists, before the disease progresses.
* To have an explanation for the symptoms you have been experiencing and to avoid the feeling that it is all psychological.
* To have the information on which to be able to make future decisions about your life, e.g. type of job, type of house, number of children etc.
* To qualify for state benefits, such as disability benefit, if MS has already affected your ability to earn a living.

WAYS OF DIAGNOSING MS

A Clinical Diagnosis

Most cases of MS are still diagnosed clinically. This means that the doctor makes the diagnosis after you have visited him or her several times, each time presenting with a different symptom. Usually, doctors wait for several different MS symptoms over a period of time – often years – before reaching a diagnosis of MS. A clinical diagnosis does not involve having tests. Some people think this method wastes precious time, waiting for patients to have further attacks before making a diagnosis.

Specific Tests For MS

Electrophoretic Mobility Test

This was devised originally by Professor E J Field as a diagnostic test, although attempts by other scientists to confirm his work have not been entirely successful. However, recent research work at Bristol Royal Infirmary has used Field's test not as a way of diagnosing MS, but as a way of testing the fatty acid content of red blood cell membranes. This test does reveal an abnormal blood lipid level in people with MS.

Another new diagnostic test for MS looks at *immunoglobulin estimations*. It has been found that there is an abnormal IgG ratio in about 54 per cent of people who have MS.

New *electrophysiology* tests can measure how long it takes from the time you stimulate a section of the nervous system using a magnetic field, to the time it reaches the target muscle. Researchers have already found that it takes longer for a message to get through in people with MS. In scientific language they call this 'an electrophysiological deficit in MS'.

Scanners

The great new hope for diagnosing MS is the use of scanners. The main types are CAT scans – Computerized Axial Tomography; NMR scans – Nuclear Magnetic Resonance; and PET scans – Positron Emission Tomography.

Scanners produce high resolution cross-sections of selected parts of the body. They are safe, comparatively non-invasive and can provide detailed information about the brain.

Scanners have the advantage of being able to 'detect' plaques and abnormalities in the brain and spinal cord. Normally, it would not be possible to invade these areas in a living person. With the aid of a scan, a doctor is able to pinpoint very specific tissue damage such as plaques, swelling, and atrophy.

As well as being able to pinpoint damage from a diagnostic point of view, scanners have a huge potential in being able to monitor the effectiveness of any treatment, by doing 'before and after' scans of patients undergoing a particular therapy.

However, the trouble with these scanners is that they are very expensive indeed and there are very few of them in the country.

At the moment they are a long way from being the standard method of diagnosis, or of confirming diagnosis of MS, or of monitoring treatments.

Standard Neurological Tests

A lumbar puncture can detect whether there is any myelin debris in the spinal fluid. This test is highly invasive and unpleasant. Many people report both short and long-term after-effects. Under local anaesthetic, a needle is inserted into the lumbar area of the spinal cord and some fluid is removed for analysis. Some people are left with a truly dreadful headache – so bad you can't lift your head off the pillow – for days afterwards.

Neurological units can also give you the *Visual Evoked Response* test, which tests your eyes. There are also tests for balance, sensation, reflexes, and other neurological signs.

The Importance of Diagnosis

If you are not happy with just a clinical diagnosis, or have not been given any diagnosis at all, ask to be referred for any or all of the above diagnostic tests. It is important to know for certain whether or not you have MS.

This book takes the view that very early diagnosis is essential, both from a practical and an ethical point of view. This is because I believe there are effective ways of controlling MS, and the sooner you start, the less likely you are to get worse. In addition, there is now some scientific evidence that taking supplements of polyunsaturated oils can stabilize MS in the recently diagnosed, (see page 60).

WHO GETS MS?

The latest estimates are that about 80,000 people in the UK have MS.

Diagnosis of MS is usually made between the ages of 20 and 40, although there are cases older and younger than this. There are more women with MS than men. The ratio is 3 to 2. No one knows exactly why this should be.

MS is much more common in temperate climates of the world. This makes Europe and North America areas high in MS, compared to continents with more tropical climates such as Asia and Africa. Hot countries, such as Israel, have a low incidence of MS among Israelis who were born there. However, if a person emigrates from Northern Europe to Israel *after* the age of 15, they carry with them the high risk of the area in which they were born and spent their childhood.

West Indians born in the UK have a similar incidence of MS to the rest of the UK population. However, the incidence of MS is low in the Caribbean. So scientists believe there may be an environmental factor involved in MS.

2

The Management of
Multiple Sclerosis

Here you are, landed with a disease with no known cause, no known cure, and no recognized treatment.

You could languish in a private hell and lament your terrible lot, or you could decide to do everything in your power to fight the disease and help yourself.

THE SELF-HELP MANAGEMENT ARMOURY

The full armoury of weapons with which to wage war on MS includes all of the following:

- Eating a healthy, low-fat diet, rich in essential fatty acids (see chapter 6).
- Supplementing your diet with essential fatty acids.
- Supplementing your diet with vitamins, minerals and trace elements.
- Testing yourself for food and other allergies and excluding substances toxic to you.
- Doing regular exercise, physiotherapy, or yoga.
- Maintaining a positive attitude to life.
- Keeping your brain active and stimulated.
- Getting enough rest.
- Avoiding fatigue.
- Leading a stress-free life, or as near stress-free as possible.
- Having satisfying relationships with other people.

- Resisting aggressive drugs which weaken the immune system.

Even if you can only manage the first three all of the time, and the others only some of the time, you would be doing a lot towards keeping yourself as fit and healthy as possible.

Make an Early Start

Start the management programme as soon as you are diagnosed. Resist being given corticosteroid drugs. The earlier you start, the better. Studies have shown that the people who benefit most from this self-help regime are the recently diagnosed. Don't wait until you get worse before you decide to try this self-help programme. Use it as an insurance policy to help prevent you from getting worse.

It is *not* a cure. It is not a recognized treatment. The best one can hope for at the moment is a *management* of the disease. It can't do you any harm and it might do you some good. It gives you a chance of enjoying life to the full – even though you have MS.

The Rationale behind this Management Programme

Having read the previous chapter, you have an idea of what is going wrong in MS. Knowing this helps explain the various objectives of the self-help management programme.

Why a Low-Fat Diet?

- Because too much saturated fat in the diet may be weakening the blood vessel walls and causing a breach of the blood–brain barrier.
- Because shifting your fat intake to polyunsaturated fats will help strengthen blood vessel walls.
- Because myelin is largely made up of lipids, i.e. polyunsaturated fats. So is the brain.
- Because in MS the central nervous system is under attack. Polyunsaturated fats are needed for the growth and repair of nervous tissue, and for the maintenance of its structure.

- Because MS is highest in those parts of the world where a lot of dairy produce is eaten, and lowest in those parts of the world where they eat more fish, and more vegetable oils.

Why Supplement Your Diet with Essential Fatty Acids?

- All of the above reasons.
- Because people with MS have abnormal red blood cells, and EFAs may help correct this.

Why Supplement Your Diet with Vitamins and Minerals?

- Because they help boost the immune system.
- Because you need certain vitamins and minerals to act as collaborators if you are eating a diet rich in essential fatty acids.
- Because your present diet may be low in them.
- Because people with MS may be low in certain vitamins and minerals, especially B6 and zinc.
- Because you need to have an optimum nutritional status to be as healthy as you can.
- Because the amalgam fillings in your teeth may be seeping tiny amounts of mercury, and certain vitamins and minerals will help to de-toxify the body.

Why Test Yourself for Food Allergies?

- Because many people with MS have allergies to certain foods.
- Because these foods are toxic to those individuals, and can make MS symptoms worse.
- You have to test yourself to see which particular foods and chemicals you are allergic to, because everyone is different.
- Many of those people with MS who have excluded the foods they are allergic to have improved as a result of doing so.

Why Do Regular Exercise, or Physiotherapy, or Yoga?

- To maintain fitness.
- To maintain suppleness and build up stamina.
- To keep maximum use of your body.
- To be able to do all your usual daily activities.
- To have more energy.
- To stop your body getting stuck in the wrong postures.
- To feel better and look better.
- To reduce anxiety and stress.
- To help calm the mind.

Why Resist Corticosteroids and Other Aggressive Drugs?

The standard treatment for attacks of MS is corticosteroid drugs. They work effectively in alleviating the symptoms of MS, and succeed well in getting people back on their feet, because they are powerful anti-inflammatory agents.

So, if they work so well, why should you not take them? These drugs *weaken* the immune system. With each course of corticosteroid drugs, the immune system is weakened still further.

The self-help management programme of a diet high in polyunsaturates plus selected vitamins, minerals and trace elements plus excluding allergenic foods does the exact opposite. Its aim is to *boost* the immune system. The more you strengthen the immune system, the more your own body can heal itself.

Herein lies the crux of the difference between the orthodox approach, and the approach taken by this book. You must choose between weakening your immune system with drugs which work well in the short term, or a nutritional therapy which will boost your immune system, but without immediate results and instant symptomatic relief.

In the long term, corticosteroid drugs also have side-effects, such as weight gain, 'moon' face, and unwanted hair. Immuno-suppressive drugs such as cyclosporin have a wide range of bad side-effects, including hypertension, swelling of the lymph nodes, and sometimes cancer.

All the other things in the self-help management programme are self-explanatory. Leading a stress-free life and avoiding fatigue are particularly important when you know how much these things can precipitate attacks.

It's a good idea to try and incorporate all these things into your normal life, rather than let them take over your life like some manic hobby. MS is a fact of life, but it is not your whole life. Don't let it take you over. Overcome it before it overcomes you.

3

The Links Between What You Eat and MS

Nutrition has had the best results so far of any kind of therapy in controlling multiple sclerosis. And the more research that is done, the more certain the benefits of nutrition become. Nutrition is an umbrella word which can include the food you eat, nutrients in the form of supplements, as well as foods to which you may be allergic, or sensitive.

These are the essential points about nutritional therapy for MS:

1. Cut down drastically on saturated fat, found in animal fats, dairy produce, and hard fats.
2. Increase your intake considerably of polyunsaturated fats. Not just in spreads and oils, but also in foods like fish, liver and green leafy vegetables. This will give you a diet high in essential fatty acids.

   Saturated fats and polyunsaturated fats work against each other in many respects. So you need to cut back on how much saturated fat you eat if you are going to increase your intake of Polyunsaturated Fatty Acids (PUFAs for short). That way, you will get maximum benefit.
3. Find out which foods and substances you personally are sensitive, or allergic, to. These may be surprisingly benign foods (e.g. apples or tomatoes), although the most common food to which MS people are allergic is milk. Cut out completely all foods and substances to which you are found to be allergic.
4. Eat a diet which gives you the best nutrition possible. Cut out junk foods and convenience foods. Always try and eat fresh

foods, rather than foods that have been processed and packaged. Cut out, or down on, foods which only give empty calories, e.g. sugar.

5. Take supplements of evening primrose oil and fish oils. This guarantees you a good intake of the essential fatty acids you need for many vital things in your body to work properly.

6. Take supplements of certain vitamins, minerals, and trace elements. Your body may be short of these and they are needed to go hand in hand with the essential fatty acids.

The next six chapters go into each of these points in detail.

The Links between Nutrition and MS

Researchers in multiple sclerosis have to be a bit like detectives. They have to search for clues, piece them together, and find the culprits.

The Geographical Distribution of MS

One of the most marked features of MS is its geographical distribution. MS is a disease of temperate zones, and is virtually non-existent in the tropics. There are obviously a great many differences between life in temperate countries and tropical countries. But the key difference seems to be the food that people eat.

In those places where MS is highest, people eat a lot of dairy produce. In those places where MS occurrence is lowest, people eat more fish and vegetable oils. The difference between an area of high MS and low MS can be as little as a few miles. So some of the starkest contrasts in MS are within Norway, comparing inland farming areas where dairy farming is practised and where MS is high, with coastal areas where people eat more fish and MS is low. There is a similar story in some Scottish islands where the rates of MS can fluctuate from very high to very low according to the main diet of the local people – high in areas of dairy farming and low in fishing areas.

Interestingly, a world map of the distribution of MS can also be interpreted in a slightly different way. The areas of high MS would also be the areas of high dental caries, which suggests that people had been eating a lot of sugar and have probably had fillings put in their teeth (see chapter 11).

One of the first doctors to look at the world map of MS was Professor Roy Swank of the USA. He first developed his famous Swank low-fat diet in 1948.

As a clever detective, Swank noticed several important clues. First, the amount of saturated fat in a typical American diet was rising dramatically. This was because there were improvements in the processing of dairy foods, beef cattle were made fatter so farmers could make more money, and processing techniques meant that vegetable oils changed from their natural states into margarines rich in saturated fat.

As the consumption of saturated fat has increased, so the incidence of certain diseases has increased – particularly MS, heart disease and strokes. A link between a high-fat diet and these diseases looked probable.

During World War II, there were more clues for any medical detectives on the look-out. It was noticed that young American soldiers who had died of heart attacks during training and battle showed a greater degree of hardening of the arteries than their Oriental counterparts who mostly ate vegetables and rice.

In occupied Norway, fat consumption fell by 50 per cent during food shortages. At the same time, there were significant reductions in death rates from heart attacks, and the rate of multiple sclerosis dropped too. But after the war, fat intake and heart disease returned to their previous rates.

As long ago as 1950, Swank wrote:

. . . possibly the incidence of the disease (MS) in entire populations may be related directly to the dietary fat – a high fat diet is not the cause of multiple sclerosis even though it may contribute to a high incidence of the disease by accelerating it in susceptible individuals.

Swank began his historical studies on low-fat diet for MS on the following hypothesis:

'The three-fold increase in fat intake in the past 200 years in the western world has caused a breakdown in the ability of the blood to maintain the fat and other matter in an emulsified state. The emulsion breaks down; the formed elements in the blood aggregate; and micro-embolism of the micro-circulation with consequent breakdown in the blood–brain barrier follow.'

In the UK, 40 per cent of our diet is saturated fat. Around the world, tipping the balance of saturated/unsaturated fat in favour of saturated fats has coincided with an increase in not just MS but also in cardiovascular (heart and stroke) diseases as well.

How Our Diet Has Changed over the Last Two Centuries

Nutritionists like Professor Michael Crawford have made a special study of how the food we eat has altered over the centuries. There have been profound changes in our diet in the last two centuries. During that time, the whole nature of the biological food chain has changed radically.

The biggest changes have been in fat and sugar. Humans used to eat meat from wild game, which was very lean meat, rich in structural fats. But since the introduction of modern farming, animals have been reared to have stores of fat, which are full of saturated fat.

The amount of sugar we eat has increased enormously in the same period of time.

Some people believe that humans were not designed to thrive on a high saturated fat plus high sugar diet. The rise in chronic diseases coincides with these radical changes in diet in the western world.

The old-fashioned way of looking at a person's nutritional needs was to divide all foods simply into the basic food groups of proteins, carbohydrates, and fats. The emphasis has been on calories and energy rather than on cellular development. It is now obvious that the typical western diet has developed the *wrong kind of fats*. What we need to do now is stop going down the wrong road, do a U-turn, and take another route.

The Composition of the Brain, the Nervous System, and Cell Membranes

The next big clue about nutrition and MS comes from a knowledge of what the brain, the nervous system, and cell membranes are made of. One of the detectives in this field has largely been Professor Michael Crawford, who has made a special study of brain growth. He devised the successful ARMS Diet in 1978.

His rationale for the low-fat diet was partly based on the MS map of the world. But it was also partly based on how the brain is put together. Roughly 60 per cent of the brain is made of structural fats. These special fats, called phosphoglycerides, are the building blocks of the central nervous system. You have to get these special fats from the diet. They are essential, and you cannot make them without eating the foods containing them. So they are called *essential fatty acids*. (These are explained in more detail in chapter 4.) Essential fatty acids are needed for the brain to work properly.

Cell membranes also need these essential fatty acids (as well as proteins) to be built properly.

Cell membranes must have fluidity and flexibility to be in good shape. They get this fluidity and flexibility from polyunsaturated fats.

So overall, the body has a great need for polyunsaturated fats. That's why a diet high in polyunsaturated fats and low in saturated fat is so important for MS.

Do People with MS have a Defect in Fats Metabolism?

Does MS develop against a background of inborn mishandling of certain essential fatty acids? This idea was the brainchild of Professor RHS Thompson of the Middlesex Hospital. This innate defect in handling fats has become known as 'Thompson's anomaly'.

Professor Thompson was first to put forward the suggestion that people with MS had a lack of certain essential fatty acids (linoleic acid and arachidonic acid) in their cell membranes. As has been said above, unsaturated fatty acids form an important constituent of the phospholipids which are a component of cell surface membranes everywhere in the body.

Other researchers did studies to see whether Thompson was right. If he was, the surface of *all cells* in the body of someone with MS would be in some way different from normal people, and from people suffering from other neurological diseases.

One of these scientists who followed on the work of Professor RHS Thompson was Professor EJ Field. He particularly studied red blood cells in MS people, and in fact devised a brilliant test which measured how fast MS red blood cells travelled in the presence of linoleic acid and arachidonic acid. This became known as the Electrophoretic Mobility Test (see page 31).

Professor Field confirmed what had been suspected: the red blood cells in people with MS are subtly different. So are the lymphocytes (white blood cells) which should play a part in the body's immune system if they are doing their job properly. This might help explain the auto-immune aspect of MS. Recent research work by Dr Rosie Jones and others at Bristol Royal Infirmary has confirmed that there is an abnormal lipid profile in the blood of people with MS, thus confirming some of Professor Field's earlier work.

The reason for nutritional therapy involving essential fatty acids is that these anomalies in cells can be corrected by eating the right foods or supplements.

4

Fats and MS

The previous chapter explained the main thinking behind why a low fat/high polyunsaturated fat diet is sensible for anyone with MS.

But before going any further, the important thing is to describe the difference between the two types of fat – saturated fat and unsaturated fat.

Saturated Fats

Saturated fats are usually hard at room temperature. Think of candles as a good example of what a hard fat looks like.

Butter, hard cheeses, and the visible fat on meat are examples of saturated fat. More subtle examples of saturated fat are in things like manufactured cakes and biscuits.

Saturated fat is not needed for any essential structures or functions of the body. Its function is to help give energy. Too much of it will be laid down in fat – the kind of 'fat' which everyone understands, spare tyres round the tummy and podge on the thighs. In short, too much padding.

Unsaturated and Polyunsaturated Fats

Generally speaking, unsaturated fats are liquid, or soft at room temperature, e.g. vegetable, seed and fish oils.

A bottle of natural sunflower seed oil, or a tub of a polyunsaturated spread such as sunflower margarine, are easy to identify as unsaturated fats. Nowadays, the word 'poly-unsaturated' is written clearly on the label of such products.

Less easy to identify are the unsaturated fats 'hidden' in foods you would not normally associate with 'fats' at all. This list includes fish, dark green leafy vegetables, offal meats such as liver, heart, kidneys, brains, lean meat, shellfish and sprouting seeds.

Whether a fat is saturated, unsaturated or polyunsaturated has to do with its biochemical composition, which is fairly complicated. The key thing to know is that polyunsaturated fats (PUFAs) are much better for people with MS than any other kind.

Fatty Acids and Essential Fatty Acids

Fat is made from smaller components called fatty acids. In biochemical terms, fatty acids are chain-like substances, some with short chains, and some with long chains. The chains are of carbon atoms with hydrogen and oxygen atoms attached. The degree of saturation depends on the extent to which they can absorb more hydrogen.

Unsaturated fats are capable of picking up other molecules available to them in the system. Saturated fats cannot take any more hydrogen.

If a fatty acid has *no* double bonds it is saturated.

If a fatty acid has *one* double bond it is unsaturated.

If a fatty acid has *two or more* double bonds it is polyunsaturated.

Figure 1 shows an example of a polyunsaturated fatty acid, linoleic acid.

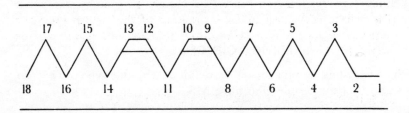

Figure 1: Linoleic Acid. This is a chain with 18 carbon atoms and two double bonds.

The body can make some of the fatty acids it needs for growth. But it is incapable of making the essential fatty acids. Essential fatty acids are called 'essential' because your body cannot make them itself. Like vitamins, essential fatty acids must be taken with the food you eat.

All essential fatty acids are polyunsaturated fatty acids (PUFAs). But the reverse is not true and not all PUFAs are essential fatty acids. In order for a PUFA to act as an EFA, highly specific chemical structures are required. The polyunsaturated fatty acid must be in what is called the 'cis' form to be biologically active.

Like certain vitamins, cis-linoleic acid and alpha-linolenic acid have no biological activity of their own, apart from being oxidized to provide energy. If they are to function as EFAs, they require specific biochemical transformation within the body. The exact functions of each of the fatty acids in the sequence (see Figure 2, page 50) are by no means fully known. However, it is known that unless cis-linoleic acid can be converted to gamma-linolenic acid (GLA) it has no biological activity as an essential fatty acid.

'Fat' is a rather misleading word to be connected with essential fatty acids. These nutrients are more like proteins, or vitamins. It is vital to eat them to stay healthy.

Essential fatty acids are present in every cell in your body, and are vital for metabolism. These are the fats which go to make up a major proportion of the brain and nervous system. This type of fat is an essential part of nutrition.

The two terms 'essential fatty acids' and 'polyunsaturated fatty acids' (PUFAs) can be confusing, since they are not necessarily the same thing. Some doctors talk about PUFAs as if they were all essential fatty acids. For simplicity's sake, whenever PUFAs are mentioned in this book they should be taken to mean those polyunsaturated fatty acids which are also essential fatty acids.

PUFAs and Multiple Sclerosis

The previous chapter looked in detail at why this type of fat is so important for people who have MS.

To recap:

- PUFAs are needed for the growth and repair of the nervous tissue.

- PUFAs are needed for the maintenance of the structure of nervous tissue. This is particularly important in MS, where the nervous system is under attack. If the body lacks these nutrients, any repair of damaged tissue is made more difficult.
- People with MS show an unusual pattern of fatty acids in their blood. With a diet rich in PUFAs, this can return to normal in between 9 months–1 year.
- Some research has shown that the white matter in the brains of people with MS is low in PUFAs.
- Perhaps people with MS have an inborn inability to handle PUFAs correctly.
- In people with MS, the myelin sheath, the red and white blood cells, the platelets, and the blood plasma are also deficient in PUFAs, particularly linoleic acid.
- PUFAs play a fundamental role in all cell membranes of the body. The fluidity and flexibility of the cell membranes depends on how much PUFAs the cells have.
- The activity of lymphocytes (white blood cells) may be dependent on the state of the cell membrane. They will behave differently according to whether a cell membrane is fluid (plenty of PUFAs) or rigid (not enough PUFAs). This influences the ability of certain lymphocytes to react immunologically.

The Families of Essential Fatty Acids

There are two families of essential fatty acids. Both families are very important to the dietary management of MS.

The first family is headed by linoleic acid. Biochemists call this the Omega 6 family, and it is often referred to like this. The other family is headed by alpha-linolenic acid. Biochemists call this the Omega 3 family.

When foods containing these two families of fatty acids are eaten, the body makes them into longer-chain, more biologically active unsaturated fatty acids. It is only these longer-chain fatty acids which are used by the brain.

The derivatives of linoleic acid and alpha-linolenic acid are more important for the brain and nervous system than the parent fatty acids. This means that gammalinolenic acid and arachidonic acid are more important than linoleic acid, and that eicosapentaenoic and docosahexaenoic acids are more important than alpha-linolenic acid.

The Derivatives of Essential Fatty Acids

It is fine to eat the parent foods, but only a small amount of the derivatives are actually produced in this way. In any case, it is thought that people with MS may not be as good as other people

FAMILY 1: *The Omega 6 family*	FAMILY 2: *The Omega 3 family*
LINOLEIC ACID Found in sunflower seeds, safflower seeds, seed oils, vegetable oils, legumes etc.	**ALPHA–LINOLENIC ACID** Found in green leafy vegetables, e.g. broccoli, spinach, kale etc, and certain legumes
↓ Addition of double bonds	
GAMMALINOLENIC ACID Found in evening primrose oil, borage oil, oats, blackcurrant oil, breast milk, etc.	
↓ Chain elongation	
DIHOMO–GAMMALINOLENIC ACID	**EICOSAPENTAENOIC ACID**
↓ Addition of double bonds	↓
ARACHIDONIC ACID Found directly in offal meats such as liver, brains, kidneys etc. Used in the nervous system	**DOCOSAHEXAENOIC ACID** Found in fish and seafood directly Used in the nervous system

Figure 2: How Longer-Chain Fatty Acids Are Made In the Body

in converting the parent essential fatty acids through to their derivatives. This is an explanation for the wonky EFA blood profile of people with MS. This means it is better to eat directly the foods containing gammalinolenic acid, arachidonic acid, eicosapent-aenoic acid and docosahexanoenoic acid.

1. Gammalinolenic Acid

Gammalinolenic acid (GLA) is 50 per cent more unsaturated than linoleic acid. It is not present in any of the commercially-produced vegetable oils. In fact, it is quite rare. The easiest way to take it is in capsules of evening primrose oil, which contain about 9 per cent GLA. It is also available in blackcurrant seed oil capsules, starflower oil (borage oil) capsules and oats. An oil with a much higher GLA content made from highly purefied borage oil is presently being researched at St Thomas' Hospital in London.

From GLA it is easy for the body to make some prostaglandins, which are vital for good health.

2. Arachidonic Acid

Arachidonic acid is one of the most important and effective of the essential fatty acids. It plays a vital role in the structure of healthy cells, and is involved in the production of prostaglandins. It may also play a part in the regulation of the body's immune system. Liver is the best and easiest source of arachidonic acid.

3. Prostaglandins

Prostaglandins may hold a vital key in the MS mystery. They are manufactured from dihomo-gammalinolenic acid and from arachidonic acid.

Prostaglandins are a newly-understood class of substance. They have a hormone-like character. Like hormones, they act as regulatory substances and as messengers. But unlike hormones, which are normally produced by one gland, prostaglandins are not produced by glands. They are produced and used very locally, as and when they are needed. They are metabolized on site, and used very quickly.

Prostaglandins have two particularly important functions to do with MS – platelet aggregation, and regulation of the immune system.

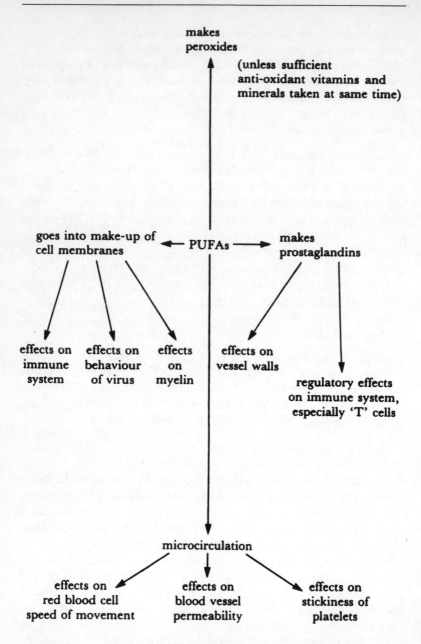

Figure 3: The various ways in which PUFAs may be working in the treatment of MS

The platelets are very small particles in the blood. They play a role in blood clotting. In MS, there is evidence to show that there is an abnormal 'clumping together' of platelets. Prostaglandins are thought to regulate the platelet functions in the blood. Using modern testing techniques, it is now possible to show that after eating a diet high in PUFAs for several months, the platelet behaviour in the blood becomes normal. It is thought that the prostaglandins, which are metabolized from certain PUFAs, play a vital role in this.

Prostaglandins and the Immune System

The other very important thing which certain prostaglandins are thought to do is regulate the immune system. Something is certainly wrong with the immune system of people with MS.

The main function of the immune system is to get rid of invading bodies, such as bacteria and viruses, from the body. MS is called an auto-immune disease. What happens is that, for some reason, the body cannot tell the difference between itself and alien things. In the confusion, the body attacks its own substances.

The kind of prostaglandins which regulate the immune system may be in short supply in people with MS. A shortage of the series 1 prostaglandins may possibly lead to defective lymphocytes, and increase the body's susceptibility to auto-immune damage (i.e. the body producing antibodies which act against its own tissues).

Prostaglandins series 1 may be of critical importance in regulating the function of some particular white blood cells involved in defending the body – the 'T' lymphocytes. One type of 'T' lymphocyte, the 'T' suppressor cells, prevent the body from attacking itself. Research has shown that levels of 'T' suppressor cells are very low in MS patients during a relapse. It is known that prostaglandins have the effect of dampening down lymphocytes which are capable of attacking the central nervous system.

So, in short, PUFAs help boost the immune system.

Possible Mechanisms by which PUFAs may be Working in MS

We have now looked at all the various reasons for eating a low fat/high polyunsaturated fat diet if you have MS.

The mechanisms which might be involved are summarized in Figure 3.

5

Recent Research on Nutrition and MS

There have been two recent studies on low saturated fat/high polyunsaturated fat diet for MS. Both come to the same broad conclusion – people with MS who stick steadfastly to a low saturated fat diet *do not get significantly worse,* whereas people with MS who do not stick to it *do* get worse.

One was done by Professor Roy Swank of the Oregon Health Sciences University in Portland, Oregon, USA.[1] The second was done by the MS Unit at the Central Middlesex Hospital in London, funded by ARMS.[2] (See end of chapter for references.)

THE SWANK RESEARCH

The most outstanding research on nutrition and MS has been carried out by Professor Roy Swank. He has championed the low saturated fat diet since 1948. His results are stark and clear-cut: MS patients who eat less than 20 grams of saturated fat a day show significantly less deterioration and much lower death rates than those MS patients who eat more than the limit of 20 grams of saturated fat a day.

His research on 144 patients spanning 34 years was published in the prestigious British journal *The Lancet* on July 7th 1990.[1] The striking results of this paper are how well the 'good dieters' did compared to the 'poor dieters'. 'Good dieters' were those who dramatically changed their former eating habits and who cut back on their saturated fat consumption to a very low level (less than

20 grams a day). 'Poor dieters' ate more saturated fat than this, sometimes two, three, or more times the limit of 20 grams a day. The lowest saturated fat consumers – who ate an average of 17g a day – showed little worsening of disability and a low death rate over the 34 years of the study; an increase in the fat intake to more than 25 grams of saturated fat a day was accompanied by a striking increase in disability and near tripling of the death rate.

When the MS patients first joined the trial they were put into one of three categories: minimum disability (initial neurological scale 1); moderate disability (initial grade 2); or severe disability (initial grades 3-5). At the end of the trial, they were assessed to see where they were on the disability scale. (See Table 1 for details of the disability scale.)

---

0 Normal performance and normal neurological findings, frequent fatigue, occasional exhaustion.

1 Normal performance physically and mentally, neurological signs present, frequent fatigue, periodic exhaustion.

2 Mildly impaired physical performance but ambulant, neurological signs present, able to work part time or full time, fatigue present and exhaustion periodic, occasional variable memory impairment.

3 Severely impaired performance but ambulant, able to work (usually part time) neurological impairment usually widespread, variable memory impairment frequently present.

4 Wheelchair needed, memory often impaired.

5 Confined to bed and chair.

6 Deceased.

Table 1: Kurtzke Neurological Disability Scale

Minimum Disability at Start of Trial (initial grade 1)

'Good dieters': 19 patients were in this category. At the end of the trial the mean neurological grade was 1.9 after 30 years on the diet.

One patient had died from MS or its complications.

'Poor dieters': Their neurological grade went up to 5.3 at the end of the trial. Four patients had died from MS or its complications.

Moderate Disability (initial grade 2)

'Good dieters': Their mean neurological grade at the end of the study was 3.6. Eight patients died from MS or its complications.

'Poor dieters': At the end of the trial their mean neurological grade was 5.4. Sixteen patients died from MS or its complications.

Severe Disability (Initial grade 3-5)

'Good dieters': By the end of the trial their mean neurological grade had changed from 3.2 to 4.0. The death rate from MS was 21 per cent.

'Poor dieters': The average neurological grade of these patients at the start of the diet was 3.2, and at completion was 5.6. 83 per cent of the patients died from MS or its complications.

In each of the three disability groups the average worsening in disability grade and the percentage of deaths of the 'poor dieters' significantly exceeded those of the 'good dieters'.

The greatest difference occurred among those who entered the study with minimum disability: 1 at the outset, compared with 1.9 for the 'good dieters' after 30 years, and 1 at the outset compared with 5.3 for 'poor dieters' at the end of the same period. This is a startling contrast, and arguably the strongest argument in this book to follow Swank's advice'

The results of this trial also showed that the sooner the low saturated fat diet is started, the greater the chance of slowing down deterioration. The greater the disability at the time of starting the diet, the lower the chances of halting deterioration.

A staggering 95 per cent of patients remained only mildly disabled after 30 years by sticking to a diet which contained less than 20 grams of saturated fat a day. This means that, thanks to changing their diet drastically, they were still able to walk, and in many cases to work, after 30 years of the disease.

Defaulting On The Diet

Professor Swank particularly warns against defaulting on the diet.

This can happen when MS patients are lulled into a false sense of security: they stick to the low saturated fat diet for a while, think their MS is under control, so assume it must be OK to cheat a little on the diet, or even drop it altogether. Herein lies the road to disaster, warns Swank.

Defaulting on the diet even after five to ten years of being on it was, in almost all cases, followed by a reactivation of the disease. Only 7 per cent of the patients who consumed more than 20g of saturated fat daily did not show a high sensitivity to fat. Swank says there is an estimated 4 per cent of MS patients who have a benign form of the disease, and this may have been the explanation as to why this small number of defaulting patients did not get significantly worse.

Professor Swank reckons that even a small increase in saturated fat can set someone rolling down the slippery slope. He noted that a saturated fat intake of 20-25 grams will not usually produce any apparent disability in a short period of time. A slow, silent deterioration occurs, and in a few years increased activity of the disease surfaces. To exceed this level repeatedly will result in the inability to lead an active life, he warns.

In recent years, Professor Swank has noticed that many patients were increasing their saturated fat intake without realizing it because they were tempted to buy new products in the supermarkets which advertised themselves as being 'low-fat' or 'no fat', or 'pure oils' when in fact they contained saturated fat.

How Much Saturated Fat is Safe?

Swank's study published in *The Lancet* is based on MS patients who ate either less than, or more than, 20 grams of saturated fat a day. It seems in that report that 20 grams was considered the safe upper limit.

However, Professor Swank's latest findings show that in fact patients consuming 10-15 grams a day of saturated fat had an even better improvement in energy and fatigue levels.

He says: 'The addition of 8 grams (1½ teaspoons) of fat often may appear to allow stabilization of the disease but this lasts for no longer than 7 years. Then the disease becomes rapidly progressive, from which there is no recovery . . . The chance that you can tolerate more than 15 grams of fat daily is no more, and probably less, than 4 per cent. Ninety-six per cent of patients who have exceeded their saturated fat by 10 grams or more have ended up deteriorating rapidly and suffered a high death rate. There is a sharp increase in disability and deaths upon the addition of 8 grams or more fat to the diet.'

Supplementation with Polyunsaturated Oils

In Swank's study, 'good dieters' consumed more oil than did the 'poor dieters' in each disability group. The oil intake of the good dieters was approximately the same as the fat intake, but the oil intake of the 'poor dieters' was significantly less than their saturated fat intake.

Swank's view is that 'the oils were beneficial to the MS patients and made it easier for them to follow the low-fat diet by broadening their choices of foods. The oils seemed to make patients feel better and increased their energy but it is doubtful that the oils were essential to their health.'

This view is not shared by some other scientists who think that the causal factor in MS is a relative deficiency of essential fatty acids, rather than a sensitivity to saturated fat. One cannot say for certain who is right. The wise decision is therefore to eat a diet very low in saturated fat which is also high in polyunsaturates.

Swank's Rationale for the Low Saturated Fat Diet

Swank believes that MS patients are very sensitive to or intolerant of saturated fatty acids, and that a high animal fat intake may be an important factor in the mechanism of the disease.

Large animal fat meals are known to cause aggregation of blood cells, slowing the circulation and reducing the amount of oxygen to the brain. This tendency to detain blood in the microcirculation could set off a complex chain of events whereby the blood–brain barrier is breached, leading to demyelination and the formation of plaques.

THE ARMS ESSENTIAL FATTY ACID DIET: RESULTS OF RESEARCH

(See chapter 6 for details of the ARMS Diet).

The results of one research study showed that the right diet does work as a treatment for MS.

Eighty-three patients with definite MS were advised to eat a diet which was low in saturated fat and high in polyunsaturated fat.

These patients were closely monitored at the MS Research Unit at the Central Middlesex Hospital for the 3-year duration of the trial. Each patient's blood was given a lipids (fats) analysis every six months.

The results of this trial are startlingly clear-cut. Patients who did not stick to the diet deteriorated significantly, whereas those who stuck faithfully to the diet did not deteriorate significantly.

The diet used in this study differed from that used in other studies on MS where only one kind of essential fatty acid – linoleic acid – had been put to the test. The intention of this diet was to decrease the amount of saturated fat, while at the same time increasing the amount of essential fatty acids of both families (linoleic and alpha-linolenic), while also providing the necessary vitamins, minerals, trace elements, and fibre.

No previous study to do with diet and MS had covered all these factors. Nor had previous studies taken into consideration the fact that EFAs compete with saturated fat. This means that when patients were not asked to restrict the amount of saturated fat they were eating, the linoleic acid on trial did not have as much chance of showing a significant result.

The conclusions of the ARMS trial are that this diet does work as a treatment as long as patients stick to it. Also, it works better, as well as being more pleasant, than drinking sunflower seed oil.

The results really leave no doubt that the ARMS Diet really works as a treatment. Doctors are urged to take heed of these findings and actually prescribe this diet as a treatment to their MS patients.

The only disappointing conclusion about this trial is that many people find it hard to stick to an optimum nutrition diet, even when they're being monitored. Unfortunately, it's all too easy to slip back into bad eating habits even when you have been instructed in new, healthier eating habits.

ARMS

Action and Research for Multiple Sclerosis was a former self-help group for MS sufferers in the United Kingdom. All the members either had MS themselves or were related to someone with MS, or had a close interest in MS. The group was founded in 1974 by a small number of people with MS who were angry that not enough was being done in the field of MS research, particularly research that might be considered as unorthodox. Membership eventually grew to several thousand. Now many of these make use of the help offered by the MS Society. (The address of the head office is in the Useful Addresses section at the end of the book.)

OTHER STUDIES ON FATS AND MS

Sunflower seed oil was first tested on MS patients in a trial conducted by leading neurologists Millar, Zilkha and others. It was written up in the British Medical Journal in 1973.[3]

The important conclusion was that the frequency, severity and duration of attacks was reduced in the group who took sunflower oil.

Starting from that time, many patients with MS began to take sunflower seed oil, either drinking it 'neat', or mixed with orange juice.

In 1978, a trial was conducted by Professor David Bates and co-workers at Newcastle University.[4] They took 116 patients with MS and divided them into four groups. Group A was given Naudicelle capsules of evening primrose oil; Group B was given capsules of olive oil; Group C was given Flora polyunsaturated margarine spread made with sunflower oil, and Group D was given a placebo spread. No advice was given regarding cutting down on saturated fats, and patients continued to eat their normal diets. Measuring the patients on a disability scale, there was no significant difference after two years between the four groups. However, they did find that the duration and severity of attacks was less severe in the group treated with Flora sunflower seed oil spread. In this group, the linoleate levels in their blood had increased by 28–39 per cent by the end of the trial period.

There was no significant elevation of linoleate in the group who were given 6 capsules of evening primrose oil a day. However, this may well be because 6 capsules a day is not sufficient to raise linoleate levels, and also because patients did not cut the amount of saturated fat, which competes with essential fatty acids. Also, at the time of this trial (1978), Naudicelle capsules contained the yellow dye tartrazine. It is now known that tartrazine inhibits the uptake of polyunsaturated fatty acids. This is another reason why the effectiveness of evening primrose oil may have been reduced in this trial. Professor Bates himself concluded that one had to take in enough polyunsaturates to affect the plasma levels of linoleate before they would have any effect on the severity and duration of relapses.

Some years after the Newcastle study, a Canadian doctor called Dr Robert Dworkin looked closely at the results of this Newcastle trial, but he pooled these results together with results from two other trials on MS and polyunsaturates. [5]

What Dr Dworkin found was very important: *Patients who had very low levels of disability at the start of the trial, who took polyunsaturates, did not get worse in a two-year period.*

This was indeed a crucial finding: The length of time that a patient had had MS made a difference to the outcome of the trials. The newly-diagnosed, who were 0-2 on the Kurtzke disability scale at the start of the trial, were the ones who showed little change or deterioration by the end of the trial. This applied only to the groups treated with polyunsaturated fatty acids.

The conclusion from this is that treatment with PUFAs helps to stabilize MS in the recently diagnosed who have no real disability. It shows that:

- There *is* a treatment for MS.
- Early diagnosis is therefore vital so that treatment can start without delay.
- If the newly-diagnosed are given polyunsaturates, they stand a good chance of stabilizing the condition.

The Fish Oil Study

Fish oils as a possible treatment for multiple sclerosis were put to the test during the 1980s, the results being published in 1989. [6] The multi-centre trial was conducted by Professor David Bates, the same consultant neurologist who conducted the 1978 Newcastle trial which looked at the effectiveness of linoleic acid.

The trial was on 312 patients with MS who were still able to walk who had the relapsing/remitting type of the disease. All the patients on the trial were given dietary advice, and recommended to increase their intake of linoleic acid. However, only half the patients were in addition given supplements of fish oils. The other half were given a placebo.

The doctors running the trial wanted to see whether the fish oil had any effect on the duration, frequency and severity of relapses. The results at the end of two years was that there was no significant improvement in the treated group, but there was a *trend in favour* of the treated group. The conclusion of the trial was, therefore, that patients with MS *should* supplement their diet with polyunsaturates from both vegetable and fish oils. Or, of course, they could eat the food sources of these two families of polyunsaturates, rather than relying on supplements.

In any case, there is now no doubt that anyone who has MS should make sure they are getting enough of both families of polyunsaturates – what scientists call omega 6 and omega 3 – better known as linoleic acid, and alpha-linolenic acid, and their derivatives.

The Future of Research into PUFAs and MS

All the indications so far are that if someone with MS takes high enough levels of polyunsaturates, both of the linoleic acid and alpha-linolenic families, while at the same time reducing saturated fats, they have a good chance of at least reducing the frequency and severity of attacks and at best of stabilizing their condition. This is more likely to be so if they start this treatment very early on in the disease, before real disability has set in.

Orthodox neurologists themselves have now proved that this is a possibility. This being so, the main thrust of new research in this field will be to test the effects of high levels of linoleate. For example, it is now possible to manufacture GLA (gammalinolenic acid) in much high quantities than the present 500mg capsules of evening primrose oil. Scientists are working on this at the moment. Among those scientists who back PUFAs for MS, there is agreement that GLA is vital, and that is why richer sources need to be developed and tested.

References

1. 'Effect of low saturated fat diet in early and late cases of multiple sclerosis'. Roy Laver Swank, Barbara Brewer Dugan. *The Lancet*, July 7 1990. Vol 336 pp 37-39.
2. 'The effect of nutritional counselling on diet and plasma EFA status in multiple sclerosis patients over 3 years'. Fitzgerald G, Harbige LS, Forti A, Crawford MA. *Human Nutrition: Applied Nutrition*, 1987; 41A 297-310.
3. 'Double blind trial of linoleate supplementation of the diet in multiple sclerosis'. Millar JGD, Zilkha KJ, Langman MJS, *et al*. *British Medical Journal*, 1973; 1:765-68.
4. 'Polyunsaturated fatty acids in treatment of acute remitting multiple sclerosis'. Bates D, Fawcett PRW, Shaw DA, Weightman D. *British Medical Journal*, 1977; ii: 1390-91.
5. 'Linoleic acid and multiple sclerosis: A reanalysis of three double blind trials'. Dworkin RH, Bates D, Millar JHD, Paty DW. *Neurology*, 1984; 34: 1441-45.
6. 'A double-blind controlled trial of long chain n-3 polyunsaturated fatty acids in the treatment of multiple sclerosis'. Bates D, Cartlidge NEF, French JM, Jackson MJ, Nightingale S, Shaw DA, Smith S, Woo E, Hawkins SA, Millar JHD, Belin J, Conroy DM, Gill SK, Sidey M, Smith AD, Thompson RHS, Zilkha K, Gale M, Sinclair HM. *Journal of Neurology, Neurosurgery and Psychiatry* 1989; 52:18–22.

6

Low Saturated Fat/High Polyunsaturated Fat Diets

A diet which is low in saturated fat and high in polyunsaturated fat is the most important part of the self-help management of MS. Research done in recent years (see previous chapter) confirms that this sort of diet can and does work if you stick to it, and should be considered a treatment for MS.

As discussed in Chapter 5, there are two main diets which are low in saturated fat and high in polyunsaturates: the ARMS EFA Diet (essential fatty acids diet) which was devised by Professor Michael Crawford; and the Swank Low Fat Diet, devised by Professor Roy Swank.

THE ARMS EFA DIET

The three main prongs of the ARMS EFA Diet are:

1. Increase the sources of essential fatty acids in the diet.
2. Cut down on saturated fat.
3. Increase intake of 'nutrient-dense' foods to meet the ARMS nutrient score targets and the NACNE (National Advisory Committee on Nutrition Education) and COMA (Committee on Medical Aspects of Food Policy) recommendations for general health.

1. Sources of Essential Fatty Acids

The sources should be from both families of essential fatty acids, linoleic and alpha-linolenic, and their long-chain derivatives – arachidonic acid, docosahexaenoic acid, and eicosapentaenoic acids.

Linoleic Acid: Oils and Margarines

Linoleic acid is found in polyunsaturated margarines and oils, e.g. sunflower, safflower, soya, sesame seed, cotton seed, corn, rapeseed, grapeseed, walnut.

Watch out for blended vegetable oils, as they are hydrogenated which means they do not contain sufficient polyunsaturates. Heating during cooking also causes hydrogenation, so avoid deep frying. Oil should only be used once, then thrown away. Once opened, store oils in the fridge.

Nuts, pulses, seeds, legumes and beans are also good sources of linoleic acid, though large amounts of nuts should not be eaten as they also contain saturated fat. Avoid coconuts and peanuts.

Arachidonic Acid: Liver, Lean Meats and Poultry

Arachidonic acid is the long-chain derivative of linoleic acid. It is found in lean meats and offal such as liver, heart, kidney, brains and sweetbreads. The ARMS diet suggests up to, but no more than, ½ lb of liver a week. Do not exceed this, as liver is high in vitamin A. You can use any kind of liver.

Shop for lean cuts of meat, and if there is any excess fat, trim this off before cooking. Go for lean pork, gammon, beef, lamb, chicken, turkey. Do not eat the skin of chicken or turkey, as this is very fatty. Game is high in arachidonic acid. This includes rabbit, venison, and partridge.

Alpha-Linolenic Acid: Green Vegetables, etc.

Alpha-linolenic acid is found in green vegetables, beans, legumes, and linseeds. The ARMS diet advises people to eat a large portion of green leafy vegetables such as broccoli, spinach, or spring greens, every day. Choose fresh or frozen, not tinned. The best way to cook vegetables is by steaming so that the nutrients are not lost.

Linseeds are available as 'Linusit Gold' from health food shops. They can be sprinkled over a variety of foods, such as breakfast cereals, salads, casseroles, etc. The other bonus of taking Linusit Gold is that it has a laxative effect. ARMS recommends a dessertspoon once a day.

At lunchtime, make it a habit to eat a raw mixed salad, with a French dressing made with a linoleic-acid oil. Include the coloured vegetables, e.g. tomatoes, carrots, beetroot, red peppers, red cabbage.

As well as being rich in minerals, vegetables – and fruit – are the best sources of vitamins C and E which protect the EFAs from damage by the air (oxidation).

Docosahexaenoic and Eicosapentaenoic Fatty Acids: Fish and Seafood

These are the long-chain derivatives of alpha-linolenic acid and are to be found in fish and seafood. The best fish are oily fish: mackerel, herring, tuna. But white fish such as cod, coley, plaice, haddock or freshwater fish such as salmon and trout are also fine. Seafood includes crab, lobster, mussels, squid, prawn, shrimps.

ARMS recommends eating fish three or four times a week. Fresh fish is best; frozen is second best; tinned is acceptable, ideally in brine.

Note: Vegetarians

It is not possible to follow the ARMS EFA diet perfectly and be a vegetarian, as the meat and fish included in the diet are considered very important. If you are a vegetarian, write to ARMS for guidance.

2. Cutting Down On Saturated Fat

This means:

* No butter.
* No lard.
* No cream.
* No full-fat cheeses.
* Cut drastically amount of medium-fat cheeses.

- No more than 3-4 eggs a week.

OK dairy produce is skimmed milk, low-fat natural yogurts, cottage cheese, curd cheese, fromage frais.

- No fatty cuts of meat.
- No meat products such as sausages, pies, pâtés.
- No shop-bought cakes, biscuits, pastries, snacks.
- No confectionery.

Instead, bake your own pastries, cakes and biscuits using wholemeal flour and polyunsaturated margarine. Instead of chocolate and sweets, which are high in saturated fat, go for fresh or dried fruit, sunflower seeds, and fruits (in moderation).

3. 'Nutrient Dense' Foods: A Wholefood Diet

The main points here are:

- Unrefined foods have more nutrients in them than refined foods. So go for wholemeal bread, cereals, pasta, brown rice. Whole grains contain the germ, and it is in the germ that essential fatty acids, vitamins, minerals and trace elements are to be found. Also, the fibre content is much higher in unrefined foods.
- Avoid sugar. If used, go for muscovado or demerara.
- Eat fresh fruit and drink fresh fruit juices – high in fibre, vitamin C and folic acid.

The ARMS Diet has been worked out so that it contains all the necessary 'co-factors' – the nutrients which the EFAs need to work with if they are to be used properly in the body. This covers a wide range of vitamins and minerals. Some of these vitamins – particularly C and E – have an anti-oxidant effect.

The ARMS nutritionists are aware that many people with MS, especially those living alone, often opt for convenience foods because it is less bother. But they urge against this as the health-giving properties of wholefoods are so much higher, and the risk of convenience foods is that they lack the essential nutrients which people with MS so badly need.

When you get hungry, the worst thing you can do is fill yourself up fast with sugar or fat-laden foods. They fill you up, but they don't have nutritive value. That's why the ARMS nutritionists advise against sugary foods or fat-laden snacks.

SUMMARY OF THE ARMS EFA DIET

1. Use polyunsaturated margarine and oils.
2. Eat at least three helpings of fish a week.
3. Eat ½ lb of liver a week.
4. Eat a large helping of dark green leafy vegetables every day.
5. Eat some raw vegetables daily, as a salad, with French dressing.
6. Eat some linseeds, or 'Linusit Gold' every day.
7. Eat some fresh fruit every day.
8. Try to eat as much fresh food as possible in preference to processed food.
9. Choose lean cuts of meat, and trim all fat away from meat before cooking.
10. Avoid hard animal fats like butter, lard, suet, dripping, and fatty foods such as cream, hard cheeses etc.
11. Eat wholegrain cereals and wholemeal bread rather than refined cereals.
12. Cut down on sugar and food containing sugar.

This diet was researched by ARMS – Action and Research for Multiple Sclerosis. Now no longer operating, ARMS was formerly a self-help group for people with multiple sclerosis and their families. The diet research was carried out at the MS Unit at the Central Middlesex Hospital.

There are a number of helpful books regarding nutritional needs and multiple sclerosis, including:

Diets to Help Multiple Sclerosis by Rita Greer, published by Thorsons.

To find out more about saturated fats and wholefood diets, readers may also want to consult:

Diets to Help Control Cholesterol by Roger Newman Turner (Thorsons).

The Fats We Need to Eat by Jeannette Ewin (Thorsons).

Healing through Nutrition by Dr Melvyn R Werbach (Thorsons).

THE SWANK LOW-FAT DIET

Full details of the Swank diet can be found in the new edition of Professor Swank's book, *The Swank Low-Fat Diet for MS*, published by Doubleday. See also page 54 for Professor Swank's latest research.

Over the years, Swank's diet has evolved to take account of new research which shows the importance of essential fatty acids. So, although his diet is still called 'the Swank Low-Fat Diet' it should really be called 'The Swank Low-Saturated Fat/High Unsaturated Fat Diet.'

In a nutshell, the Swank diet has the following guidelines:

- Oils containing essential fatty acids must be included in the quantity of at least 20g (4 teaspoonfuls) a day. Working, walking people could increase this to 8 teaspoonfuls, and very active people could take 10 teaspoonfuls.
- Exclude all dairy products and all processed foods containing hidden fat.
- Fat in meat, poultry, liver and eggs must be kept down to a minimum. The maximum saturated fat allowed is 3 teaspoons a day. *No red meat at all* should be eaten in the first year.

Foods Containing Essential Fatty Acids

- Sunflower seed oil, safflower seed oil, soybean oil, corn oil, linseed oil, cod liver oil, oil of evening primrose.
- Polyunsaturated margarines.
- Tuna fish, salmon, sardines, herring, mackerel.

- Sunflower seeds, sesame seeds, peanuts (and peanut butter as long as it is not hydrogenated), almonds, cashew nuts.
- Dark green leafy vegetables, such as spinach.

Foods Allowed in Any Quantity

These foods contain no, or very little, saturated fat:

- Eggs, whites only.
- White fish, any kind.
- Shellfish, any kind.
- Breast of poultry with skin removed.
- Skimmed milk.
- Low-fat cottage cheese.
- Low fat yogurt.
- 99 per cent fat-free cheese.
- Clear soups; beef or chicken broth; bouillon; consommé.
- Wholemeal bread.
- Matzos.
- Whole-grain cereals.
- Rice.
- Pasta.
- Corn meal.
- All fresh fruit.
- All fresh vegetables (cook vegetables with steamer or eat raw).
- Frozen or canned vegetables without butter.
- Jam and marmalade.
- Honey.
- Sugar, molasses, treacle, maple syrup.
- Jelly.
- Tea, coffee.
- Carbonated drinks.
- Alcoholic drinks in moderation.

Moderately Allowed Saturated Fat Foods

The maximum saturated fat allowed per day is 3 teaspoons. The largest simple source of fat in our diet is meat.

Table 2: Fat Content of Food

Food	Amount equal to 1 teaspoonful of fat
Eggs	1 whole
Chicken gizzards	3 oz (90g)
Chicken livers	3 oz (90g)
Heart: calf's, beef	3 oz (90g)
Kidney: pork, veal, lamb	3 oz (90g)
Leg of lamb	3 oz (90g)
Liver: beef, calf or pork	3 oz (90g)
Tongue: calf	3 oz (90g)
Beef, lean	2 oz (60g)
Chicken and turkey – dark meat, skin removed	2 oz (60g)
Chicken and turkey hearts	2 oz (60g)
Heart: lamb	2 oz (60g)
Ham, lean	2 oz (60g)
Kidney: beef	2 oz (60g)
Lamb: rib, loin, shoulder	2 oz (60g)
Pheasant, skin removed	2 oz (60g)
Pork, lean	2 oz (60g)
Rabbit	2 oz (60g)
Tongue: beef	2 oz (60g)
Veal	2 oz (60g)
Bacon	1 oz (30g)
Duck	1 oz (30g)

Forbidden Foods

- Whole milk, cream, butter, sour cream, ice cream, natural and processed cheese of any kind, all imitation dairy products (often contain palm oil which is saturated fat).
- All hard margarines, shortening, lard, chocolate, cocoa butter, coconut, coconut and palm oil.

- All packaged commercial mixes for cakes, biscuits, etc. Potato crisps, party-type snacks. All commercially prepared pies, cakes, pastries, doughnuts, biscuits.
- All processed meat and poultry, luncheon meat, salami, frankfurters, all sausages, canned meat products.
- Tinned foods which contain cream, meat, or dairy produce.

General Guidelines to the Swank Diet

Ideally, eat fresh foods. If you buy anything in tins or packets, read the label carefully. If any product does not specify the kind of vegetable oil used, avoid it.

Weigh food after it has been cooked, not before.

Use only wholegrain products, e.g. wholemeal bread, brown rice, wholewheat spaghetti, etc.

Although this is not a vegetarian diet, most protein should be taken from foods other than red meat. At least five days a week, you should get your protein from eggs, fish, seafood, skinned chicken, or turkey breast. Fish contains as much protein and amino acids as meat, and is an important part of this diet.

The fat and oil intake should be distributed over the course of the day. Eat three or four meals of about the same size, rather than snacks here and there and a heavy meal at the end of the day.

When eating out, avoid creamed foods, gravies and sauces. Avoid fried foods, including chips. Avoid foods cooked in butter and cream. Avoid puddings, except fruit salad.

Chinese and Japanese food is generally low in saturated fat and high in unsaturated fat – except spare ribs, duck, and deep-fried dishes.

If you are asked out to a dinner party, it is wise to warn your host in advance about your diet.

Lifestyle

Professor Swank publishes a monthly newsletter which goes into various aspects of living, such as advice about what to do in hot weather. He is particularly keen that his low-fat diet should be combined with adequate rest. Physical and mental fatigue must be avoided. Patients are instructed to rest a minimum of one hour a day, ideally lying down after lunch.

Professor Swank's newsletter is obtainable from:

The Swank MS Foundation
13655 SW Jenkins Road
Beaverton
Oregon 97005
USA

Conclusion

There are many similarities between the ARMS EFA Diet and the Swank Diet. The starting off point for the ARMS diet was high polyunsaturates; the starting off point for Swank's diet was low saturated fat. Each has met half way in that the ARMS diet recognizes the importance of decreasing the intake of saturated fat while increasing the intake of polyunsaturates, whereas the Swank diet has evolved to give more and more importance to increasing polyunsaturates while decreasing saturated fat.

The main point of difference is that the ARMS EFA diet strongly recommends lean meat, whereas meat is excluded in the Swank diet for the first year.

You must choose which one you prefer. The important thing is to change your diet so that it is basically high in polyunsaturates and low in saturated fat; healthy; and nutritious. The evidence so far shows that it *does* make a difference.

7

Supplements 1: Evening Primrose Oil and Fish Oils

WHY TAKE SUPPLEMENTS?

The main reason for taking supplements is because you may be deficient in certain nutrients and by taking supplements you will correct the deficiency. Many people with MS are thought to have problems with absorbing certain nutrients. Another good reason for taking all the supplements described here is because they *boost the immune system*.

Not everybody agrees that you need to take supplements. ARMS, for example, in its book on the ARMS EFA diet, says: 'Supplements in the form of vitamins, minerals and oils should not be necessary. The "Essential Fatty Acid Diet", when followed carefully, will provide adequate amounts of all the nutrients.'

The other reason why Professor Crawford is against supplements is that he is trying to encourage people to eat a diet of optimum nutrition, and he fears that taking supplements will make people eat less nutritious food. He says, 'The basic principle is to meet targets set for different fatty acids using *food* rather than pills and supplements. Experience tells us that people who rely on supplements tend to ignore food which means the nutrients not covered by the supplement suffer.' Although I basically agree with Professor Crawford's statement, I nevertheless think that there are good and justifiable reasons for people with MS to take supplements.

Firstly, the key phrase about the ARMS diet is '*when followed carefully*'. Results of a 3-year study conducted by ARMS showed that about a third of those MS people given dietary advice did *not* follow it. These were described in the results as 'non-compliers', and were the ones who got worse.

Although in theory it might be hoped that everyone would stick to a healthy diet for their own good, the evidence does not back this up. It is notoriously difficult to change one's eating habits dramatically. It is sometimes possible to do this for a short time if you are very highly-motivated, but it is hard to keep it up. Again, the results of the ARMS study showed that people were keenest to improve their nutrition in the first six months but after that improvements levelled off, even though there was still room for improvement.

Supplements seem to be absolutely vital for the people who are simply *not* going to stick to a good diet, however hard you try and persuade them to.

But there are other reasons, too, why everyone with MS would do well to take supplements, not just the 'non-compliers' on the diet. Supplements such as evening primrose oil contain a substance called gammalinolenic acid (GLA) which one cannot get from any commonly available food. It is possible for the body to make gammalinolenic from linoleic acid, but this conversion step is thought to be somewhat blocked in people who have MS, and in some other people too.

The derivatives of GLA are particularly important, as it is from GLA that prostaglandins series 1 are produced. These are described in more detail below.

The emphasis of the ARMS Essential Fatty Acid diet is very much to make arachidonic acid, and that is why liver is promoted so strongly on the ARMS diet. However, a derivative of arachidonic acid, prostaglandins series 2, may not be so good for you as the prostaglandins series 1, which are manufactured easily from evening primrose oil, but with more difficulty from foods containing linoleic acid.

Another good reason for supplementing is that the nutrient target levels set by the ARMS diet (see page 64) are above the recommended daily allowances, although not by a great deal. There is therefore a case to be made for taking certain vitamins and minerals in far higher amounts than those targeted for in the ARMS diet. Taking supplements is the only way to get these larger amounts of vitamins and minerals. This will be discussed in detail in the next chapter on vitamin and mineral supplements.

EVENING PRIMROSE OIL

The oil comes from the evening primrose plant. In recent years, this plant has gone through a metamorphosis. It used to be just a humble wild flower growing along roadsides and railway tracks or on sand dunes. Now it is also a crop which farmers cultivate and harvest on a growing scale in many countries of the world. The passage of the evening primrose from wild flower to cash crop is largely because of the medicinal potential of its oil.

There are many different types of evening primrose plant. Usually, the petals are a primrose-like yellow, and the flowers only open in the evenings. Strangely enough, the plant is not one of the primrose family at all, but belongs to the rose-bay willow-herb family.

In 1949, the seeds of the evening primrose plant were analysed using modern techniques. They were found to contain a high percentage of linoleic acid plus the very rare gammalinolenic acid. GLA is much more biologically active than linoleic acid.

In recent years, new sources of GLA have been discovered. However, these may not be as effective as evening primrose oil (see page 91).

Evening Primrose Oil and Multiple Sclerosis

Thanks to the work of scientists like Professor RHS Thompson, Professor Roy Swank and Professor Hugh Sinclair, doctors working in the field of Multiple Sclerosis thought it was worth investigating further the link between unsaturated fats and multiple sclerosis.

The first big trial to do with linoleic acid and MS was done in 1973 by Dr JHD Millar of Belfast and Dr KJ Zilkha of the National Hospital in London, and others. They found that when linoleic acid, in the form of sunflower seed oil, was given to patients with MS it reduced the frequency and severity of relapses.

After that, sunflower seed oil in various forms became all the rage with MS patients. They drank it neat, they took it in emulsions, they mixed it with orange juice. Many of them didn't like it.

At this time, evening primrose oil capsules were already being manufactured by one company only, Bio-Oil Research Ltd, of

First stages of growth

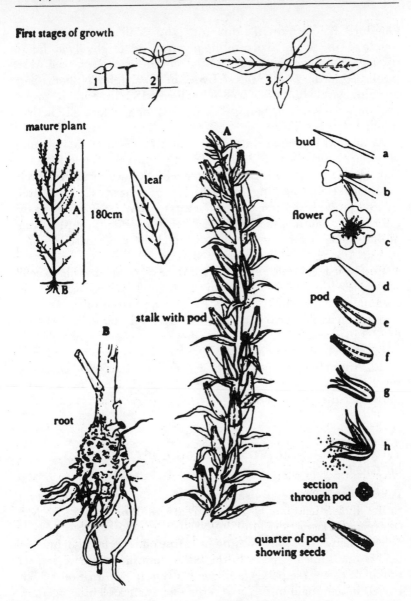

Figure 4: The Evening Primrose plant (Oenothera biennis)

The Evening Primrose plant (*Oenothera biennis*). 1–3, young plants with 2, 4 and 6 leaves; a–h, stages in development of flower, pod and seeds. *By kind permission of Rita Greer.*

Cheshire. It was Bio-Oil's director, John Williams, who was the first to see the potential of evening primrose oil, originally for heart disease. But when the results of the sunflower seed oil trial were published in the *British Medical Journal* in 1973, John Williams had a brainwave. If sunflower seed oil helped MS a little, then surely, evening primrose oil, being that much more biologically active, might help even more.

At around the same time, Professor EJ Field was doing some very important research work on essential fatty acids and MS. He started this research while Director of the Medical Research Council's Demyelinating Diseases Unit in Newcastle and later carried on with the research at Newcastle University, funded by ARMS (at that time the Multiple Sclerosis Action Group). It was at this time that I first met Professor Field and was advised by him to start taking 'Naudicelle' immediately.

Professor Field tested evening primrose oil on the red blood cells of people with MS. The results of these blood tests proved that the gammalinolenic acid (GLA) in evening primrose oil was much better than linoleic acid in correcting the defects found in the blood of MS patients.

I was one of the MS patients whose blood was tested by Professor Field. After almost a year of taking evening primrose oil capsules, my EFA blood abnormalities were corrected. I was not on any particular diet at the time.

Why Evening Primrose Oil is Better than Linoleic Acid

It has already been established that essential fatty acids belonging to the linoleic acid family (omega 6) are vital for people with MS (see page 49).

The main reason why evening primrose oil is better than linoleic acid is that the conversion in the body from linoleic acid (step 1) to the next stage (step 2) is inefficient. Evening primrose oil, which is rich in gammalinolenic acid, cuts out this problem altogether. After step 2, there are no problems in converting essential fatty acids into their derivative, in this case prostaglandins series 1. Evening primrose oil starts at step 2.

There are a number of reasons why the conversion of linoleic acid to gammalinolenic acid is inefficient, not just in people with

MS but in others too. This particular stage of the metabolic pathway is fraught with possible road blocks, or blocking agents.

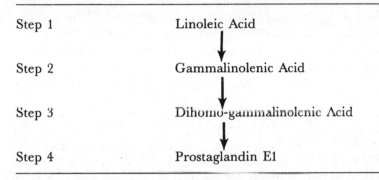

Step 1	Linoleic Acid
Step 2	Gammalinolenic Acid
Step 3	Dihomo-gammalinolenic Acid
Step 4	Prostaglandin E1

Figure 5: The normal metabolic pathway of linoleic acid.

Blocking Agents

These are the most common blocking agents:

- Foods rich in saturated fat.
- Foods rich in cholesterol.
- Too much sugar.
- Alcohol in moderate to large amounts.
- Zinc deficiencies.
- The stress hormone cortisol, rampant in situations of 'helplessness and hopelessness'.
- Viral infections.
- Radiation.
- Cancer.
- Ageing.
- Diabetes.

With this information, the metabolic pathway of linoleic acid takes on a different picture.

Co-Factors

As can be seen from Figure 6, the process of chain elongation needs certain vitamins, minerals, and trace elements (see next chapter). The important co-factors between step 1, Linoleic Acid and step

STEP 1:   CIS-LINOLEIC ACID

                 ↓

                 Enzyme delta 6–desaturase
                 needed to get to step 2

                 helped by↓
                 zinc, magnesium, vitamin B6, biotin

                 ↓

                 BLOCKED BY SATURATED FATS

                 BLOCKED BY CHOLESTEROL

                 BLOCKED BY TOO MUCH ALCOHOL

                 BLOCKED BY TOO LITTLE ZINC

                 BLOCKED BY TOO MUCH CORTISOL

                 BLOCKED BY VIRAL INFECTIONS

                 BLOCKED BY TOO MUCH SUGAR

                 BLOCKED BY CHEMICAL CARCINOGENS

                 BLOCKED BY IONIZING RADIATION

                 BLOCKED BY AGEING

                 ↓

STEP 2:   GAMMALINOLENIC ACID
                 (Evening primrose oil starts here)

                 ↓

STEP 3:   DIHOMO–GAMMALINOLENIC ACID

                 ↓

                 helped by vitamin C, vitamin B3 (nicotinic acid)

                 ↓

STEP 4:   PROSTAGLANDIN E1

Figure 6: The Bumpy Metabolic Road of Cis-Linoleic Acid

2, Gammalinolenic Acid (GLA) are vitamin B6, biotin, zinc and magnesium.

GLA and Prostaglandins

Evening primrose oil has an enormous head start on linoleic acid because it begins its journey at step 2, GLA, and never has to get over the obstacles in the path between step 1 and step 2.

GLA, though important in itself, is also a precursor of something that is vitally important – the prostaglandins series 1.

The GLA in evening primrose oil will convert easily into prostaglandins 1. This takes a different route from foods containing arachidonic acid, e.g. liver, which go on to make prostaglandins series 2. There is some disagreement amongst scientists as to whether the EFAs eaten should favour arachidonic acid (as in the ARMS diet) or prostaglandins 1 (those in favour of taking evening primrose oil). In this debate, I back those scientists who favour taking evening primrose oil. It would be fair to say there is no hard and fast evidence to back either approach.

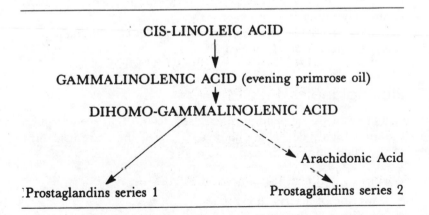

Figure 7: The Precursors to Prostaglandins 1 and 2.

Prostaglandins in general are vital cell regulators. They control every cell and every organ in your body on a second-by-second basis. The nearest thing to them is hormones, which also have important messenger roles. But prostaglandins aren't like hormones, which zip around all over the place. Prostaglandins are much more local than that. So they're a bit like friendly neighbourhood hormones, regulating everything only on their home patch.

Each prostaglandin has a very specific effect in each tissue. Generally, prostaglandins help to control what each and every cell is doing, and they regulate the activity of certain key enzymes. Prostaglandins have a very short life span. Most prostaglandins are removed from the blood during a single passage through the lungs.

Types of Prostaglandins

There are three series of prostaglandins – PG1, PG2, and PG3. Each of these has a different chemical structure, and just to make things more complicated, within each series there are many types of PGs, such as A, B, D, E, F, etc. In all, there are at least 30 prostaglandins.

In humans, the three series of prostaglandins are each derived from a different fatty acid. Series 1 and 2 both come from the linoleic acid family. Series 3 PGs are from eicosapentaenoic acid, a member of the alpha-linolenic acid family, which is most commonly found in oily sea foods.

Evening primrose oil, whose active ingredient is gammalinolenic acid, is a precursor of series 1 PGs.

Prostaglandins 1 (PGE1)

Out of all the prostaglandins researched so far, PGE1 seems to have the most highly desirable qualities. In brief, these are just some of the good things it is responsible for:

• Dilation of blood vessels.
• Lowering of arterial pressure.
• Inhibition of thrombosis.
• Inhibition of cholesterol synthesis.
• Inhibition of inflammation.
• Activation of defective T-lymphocytes.
• Inhibition of platelet aggregation.

It's worth stressing again that PGE1 is derived from gammalinolenic acid, which is the active ingredient of evening primrose oil.

This particular prostaglandin is *not* derived from eating lean meat or liver, or any of the foods rich in arachidonic acid.

In fact, arachidonic acid has as its derivative the series 2 prostaglandins which, by comparison with PG1, are more involved in inflammatory processes.

My own opinion is that it is because evening primrose oil goes on to make prostaglandin series 1 that it should be taken as a supplement in addition to eating a low-fat/high polyunsaturated fat diet.

How Evening Primrose Oil Might Be Working in MS

It stimulates the T-lymphocytes (i.e. it boosts the immune system)

Prostaglandin E1 stimulates the normal function of 'T' suppressor lymphocytes. These are white blood cells which keep the other parts of the immune system under control and which make sure that the body's defences attack foreign materials and not the body's own tissues. When 'T' suppressor cells are defective, auto-immune damage frequently occurs. Research has shown that 'T' suppressor cells are very low in MS patients during a relapse, the prostaglandin E1 may help prevent this.

It is known that PGE1 has the effect of dampening down the B lymphocytes which are capable of attacking the central nervous system.

It stops the platelets clumping together

In MS there is evidence to show that the platelets clump together in an abnormal way. The platelets are the small plate-like particles in the blood which help the blood clot. PGE1 regulates the platelets and stops them bunching up together, sticking to each other, and to blood vessel walls.

It makes faulty red blood cells return to normal

In MS, red blood cells are not only very low in essential fatty acids, they are also much bigger than they ought to be, are abnormally shaped, and have a poor ability to regulate the passage of fluids through cell membranes. Evening primrose oil can correct this defect within a matter of months.

Evening primrose oil has also been shown to correct the defect in the mobility of red blood cells. Electrophoretic mobility tests have shown that the red blood cells of people with MS move more slowly than those of healthy people. After several months of evening primrose oil supplements, these red cells have been shown to behave normally.

In a recent follow-up study of MS patients on long-term treatment with evening primrose oil ('Naudicelle'), who were also following a diet low in saturated fat, it was found that the mobility of the red cells returned to normal. The most responsive cases were those who had experienced frequent relapses.

It strengthens blood vessel walls

Prostaglandin E1 is known to strengthen blood vessel walls. This is particularly important in MS because there is growing evidence that in the microcirculation of people with MS, the blood vessel walls are breached so that blood – which is toxic to nerve tissue – seeps into the brain. By strengthening the blood vessel walls, the walls are also better able to withstand things like platelets and cholesterol from clumping together and sticking to them.

Some people believe that partly-digested food is able to get through the intestine walls in people with MS, which may be a factor in food allergies. PGE1 may help here too.

It possibly acts as an anti-viral agent

When human cells become transformed by viruses, they always lose the ability to convert linoleic acid to gammalinolenic acid, and so can't make PGE1. This may make the transformed cells resistant to attack by the body's natural defences, the immune system. Evening primrose oil gets over this problem by its ability to convert easily into PGE1. PGE1 may restore the cells' normal susceptibility to the body's immune system.

It affects the nervous system

Prostaglandin E1 has effects on nerve conduction and on the action of nerves. This can produce profound changes in the workings of both the central nervous system and the peripheral nervous system. PGE1 has strong regulating effects on the release of neurotransmitters at nerve endings and also on the post-synaptic actions of the released transmitters.

It maintains a healthy balance between the 1 and 2 series prostaglandins

If the body is very low in essential fatty acids, there is a sharp rise in the 2 series PGs, which are made from arachidonic acid. A high level of the 2 series PGs is a feature of various inflammatory disorders, such as rheumatoid arthritis and probably multiple sclerosis. It has recently been shown that the cerebrospinal fluid from MS patients contains high levels of PGF2 alpha.

Once you increase the amount of essential fatty acids in the diet, PGE1 is back on the scene. Enough PGE1 means that there is a healthy balance in the amount of 1 and 2 series prostaglandins being produced.

Another thing that evening primrose oil does is that it makes it

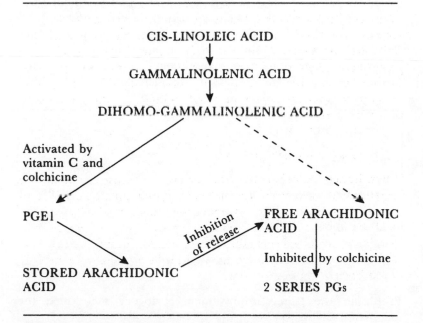

Figure 8: How Evening Primrose Oil Favours the PGE1 Route

more likely that PGE1 will be produced, as against PG2. At the junction where the road forks at dihomo-gammalinolenic acid, it persuades the traveller to follow the route towards PGE1 instead of taking the route towards arachidonic acid and the 2 series PGs (see Figure 8).

REPORTED BENEFITS OF EVENING PRIMROSE OIL ON MS

Many of the reported benefits of evening primrose oil are anecdotal – numerous personal stories told either by letter or word of mouth. Obviously, this is not scientific evidence and will not be good enough for hard scientists. But this wealth of anecdotal evidence will be heartening to people who actually have MS.

During 1979, a survey was carried out by Bio Oil Research Ltd to assess the views of MS patients taking 'Naudicelle' as a dietary supplement. Out of 480 MS sufferers taking part in the survey, 65 per cent felt there was some improvement in their condition. Of these, 43 per cent said there had been a stabilization of their condition (they had got no better, but they had got no worse); 22 per cent said there had been fewer and less severe attacks; 20 per cent said certain symptoms had been alleviated; 13 per cent reported an improvement in general health; 2 per cent reported further beneficial side-effects. The overall results look like this:

Some improvement	65%
No change	22%
Deteriorated	10%
Don't know	3%

Improvements

People in the 'some improvement' category mentioned the following benefits:

- Increased mobility.
- Increased walking ability.
- Reduced spasm or tremor.
- Improved bladder function.
- Improved eyesight.
- Improved condition of hair and skin.
- Relief of constipation.
- Improvement in wound healing.
- Regaining correct weight.
- Heavy periods returned to normal.

Note: The 'improved' group contained a significantly higher proportion of MS patients who had been diagnosed within the preceding four years.

The ARMS Survey

In 1977, ARMS sent out a questionnaire to all its members to find out what effect 'Naudicelle' was having on them. They were also asked to get an opinion from their own GP as to their condition since taking the capsules. These were the results of the 177 completed questionnaires returned:

Improved	127
No change	33
Worse	17

Of the 127 in the 'improved' category, there were 59 testimonials from GPs supporting this assessment. (Not everybody who filled in the questionnaire bothered to see their doctor.)

Even though this survey has no scientific standing, and all the answers are based only on the subjective opinions of the MS sufferer who filled in the questionnaire, the results were nevertheless extremely encouraging.

ARMS members were also asked how long they had been taking 'Naudicelle'. The answers showed that improvements increased when they had been taking the capsules for more than four months. Beneficial effects appeared as follows:

Duration of capsule use	Percentage reporting beneficial effects
Under 4 months	35%
4 months to 1 year	73%
1 to 2 years	73%
2 to 3 years	82%

At the time of the survey, very few members had been on 'Naudicelle' for longer than three years.

Of the people who returned the completed questionnaires, 141 were also on some kind of diet. The results showed that the people who were on a low saturated fat diet had better results with the evening primrose oil.

Clinical Trials on Evening Primrose Oil and MS

Two clinical trials involving evening primrose oil took place in Newcastle in 1978, conducted by Professor David Bates and others. These are described on page 60.

The researchers divided 116 people with MS into 4 groups. One group was given evening primrose oil, 'Naudicelle' 6 capsules a day; one group was given olive oil in capsules; one group was given 'Flora' to eat as a spread; one group was given another spread. (No one knew what they were taking.) At the end of the two years, there was no significant difference between any of the groups, as measured by the Kurtzke disability scale.

Of all the groups, those who did best were the ones who took the sunflower seed oil spread 'Flora'. The duration and severity of their attacks were less severe. In this group, the amount of linoleate in their blood went up from 28 per cent before the trial started to 39 per cent at the end of the trial.

Professor Bates came to the conclusion that the amount of polyunsaturates taken has to be enough to affect plasma levels. Only when this level has been achieved does the PUFA have an effect on the severity and duration of relapses.

The results of this trial are sometimes taken to prove that evening primrose oil does not work. This is not a fair assessment at all. What the trial results do show is that six capsules of evening primrose oil on their own without any additional intake of linoleic acid is not enough to affect plasma levels of linoleate.

Some people have criticized this particular trial on two counts. Firstly, that there was no advice given about cutting down on saturated fats in the diet. Saturated fats are thought to compete with polyunsaturated fats. Secondly, the 'Naudicelle' capsules used at that time had orange and black coloured shells which used the dye tartrazine. It is known that tartrazine interferes with fatty acid metabolism. Since then, evening primrose oil capsules have been produced in clear gelatin shells, with none of the same problems.

In everyday life, you are likely to eat a good amount of linoleic acid in addition to taking 6 capsules of evening primrose oil. This would be in the form of a sunflower seed oil margarine, cooking oils such as sunflower or safflower seed oil, and oils rich in linoleic acid for salad dressing.

However, it is a pity that no one has conducted another trial involving evening primrose oil taking these factors into consideration.

Since there has been no scientific evidence in favour of evening primrose oil as a therapy for MS, it is not prescribable on the NHS and has to be bought from chemists or health food shops, or by mail order from the manufacturers. Many people with MS find evening primrose oil too expensive to buy, and don't take it at all. (Discounts are possible. See page 263.)

Note: All these studies took place before Efamol or other brands were available on the market.

FISH OILS (SOMETIMES CALLED MARINE OILS)

In the last few years, the spotlight has fallen on the importance of the alpha-linolenic family of essential fatty acids. The richest source of alpha-linolenic acid is oily seafoods.

It is now believed that the best way to take essential fatty acids is a balance of the linoleic acid family and alpha-linolenic family. Scientists disagree on the ideal ratio. Some say 1:1; others 3:1

(linoleic acid to alpha-linolenic acid); others 5:1. Until this is resolved, it seems sensible to go for a happy medium.

There is nothing very new about research into fish oils. More than 30 years ago, the late Professor Hugh Sinclair had understood that the reason why Eskimos did not get the chronic diseases of western civilization was because their intake of fish oils was so high. The type of fat which comes from fish oils is used in the brain and nervous system. That old wives' tale that fish is good for your brain is actually true! It is eicosapentanoeic acid together with arachidonic acid, and not linoleic acid, which is used in the brain.

Many evening primrose oil capsules are now produced in combination with a variety of fish oils. If you buy an evening primrose oil product on its own, it is important to make sure you are taking enough fish oils, or alpha-linolenic acid in another form, e.g. linseeds or 'Linusit Gold'.

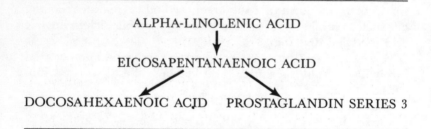

Figure 9: Alpha-Linolenic Acid Turns into Longer-Chain Fatty Acids and From Then to Prostaglandins Series 3

Fish Oil Capsules

A good supplement of fish oils is MaxEpa, or cod liver oil capsules.

Vitamin E

It is absolutely vital that you take vitamin E at the same time as taking evening primrose oil. The vitamin E acts as an anti-oxidant. Without anti-oxidants, PUFAs can create harmful peroxides (see 'free radicals' on page 96).

Many evening primrose oil capsules contain vitamin E. Some of the cheaper brands do not. So if you buy a brand which is without vitamin E, be sure to take a supplement of vitamin E. (See chapter 8 on vitamins and minerals.)

Co-Factors

In order for evening primrose oil to be metabolized properly, it needs to be taken with the following vitamins and minerals:

Vitamin C
Vitamin B6
Vitamin B3 (better known as nicotinic acid or niacin)
Zinc
Magnesium

These are described in more detail in the next chapter.

Boosting the Immune System

All these nutrients, taken together, have the effect of boosting the immune system. This is in contrast to drugs such as steroids which, although they have short-term success in their anti-inflammatory action, in the long term they *weaken* the immune system.

Other Sources of GLA (Gammalinolenic acid)

In recent years, new sources of GLA have been found. These are blackcurrant seed oil, borage oil, and GLA derived from a fermentation process which produces a fungal oil. GLA has also been found to be present in oats. The manufacturers of these newer sources of GLA claim that their GLA content is higher than evening primrose oil.

For example, one manufacturer of blackcurrant seed oil claims that the GLA content of 'Glanolin' is 17 per cent, whereas the GLA content of evening primrose oil is approximately 9 per cent. The manufacturers of the GLA derived from mould claim their GLA content is 14–16 per cent. Borage oil is thought to contain 18–20 per cent GLA.

Both blackcurrant seed oil and borage seed oil also contain some fatty acids which are not present in evening primrose oil. It is not known whether these unusual fatty acids might interfere with the action of GLA, so a higher content of GLA does not necessarily mean a better effect.

A doctor in Sweden who has MS herself and who runs an MS clinic has found blackcurrant seed oil to be less good than evening primrose oil.

However, it is too early to reach a conclusion about these higher sources of GLA. For the moment, evening primrose oil is the source of GLA which has been most tried and tested for multiple sclerosis.

'Superoil'

At the time of writing, research is underway on a 'superoil' which will contain GLA at much higher doses than that found in evening primrose oil, together with a fish oil in a compatible ratio, plus other essential fatty acids such as oleic acid. It is worth keeping your eyes open for when this product may come on the market.

8

Supplements 2: Vitamins, Minerals, Trace Elements and Amino Acids

There are good reasons to take supplements of vitamins and minerals. Firstly, your diet may not be providing enough. Secondly, you may need more than a normal person because you have a chronic illness. Thirdly, some specific vitamins and minerals are vital for the biochemical conversion process of essential fatty acids. And lastly, certain vitamins and minerals are essential if you are taking EFAs, to prevent them from oxidation.

Doctors like to tell you that you will be getting enough vitamins and minerals 'if you are eating a balanced diet'. This may not be true for people with MS.

ARMS say that supplements of vitamins and minerals are not necessary *if you stick* to their EFA diet, which is high in all nutrients including vitamins and minerals. But, as with all diets, many people do *not* stick to them, human frailty being what it is. In their own research, ARMS found that more than a third of people with MS on their study did not comply with the dietary advice given.

In an ideal world, one would eat nutritionally optimum food all the time and this would be a good source of vitamins and minerals. It is a worthy aim, and I am all in favour of optimum nutrition – I do not believe that supplements should be taken *instead* of eating a healthy diet. It is interesting to see that a recent survey in the USA found that 60 per cent of professional nutritionists, who should know how to eat, regularly took nutritional supplements.

My own view is that taking supplements of vitamins and minerals is a sensible insurance policy to be absolutely sure you are getting enough of them.

Doctors specializing in nutritional medicine, who have the equipment to do accurate nutritional profiles, find that, typically, someone with MS is deficient, sometimes grossly deficient, in vitamin B12, vitamin B1, magnesium and zinc.

Some of the doses in supplements would be much higher than normally found in foods (e.g. vitamin C). The doses recommended in this book for supplements are all higher than the target levels for dietary nutrients set by ARMS.

The following vitamins, minerals and trace elements are especially important. The reasons for taking each of them will be explained.

Vitamins

Vitamin B1
Vitamin B6 (also known as pyridoxine)
Vitamin B3 (also known as niacin, nicotinamide or nicotinic acid)
Vitamin B12
Biotin (one of the B vitamins)
All the other B vitamins
Vitamin C
Vitamin E

Minerals and Trace Elements

Zinc
Magnesium
Manganese
Molybdenum
Selenium
Vanadium

Phospholipids

Lecithin

The above list is of course in addition to evening primrose oil or other form of GLA, plus fish oils as described in the previous chapter.

THE CO-FACTORS NEEDED FOR EFA SYNTHESIS

A reminder of the metabolic pathway of EFAs (Figure 10) shows just where certain vitamins and minerals are needed to help the process along.

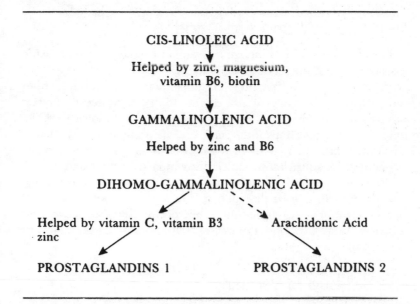

CIS-LINOLEIC ACID

Helped by zinc, magnesium,
vitamin B6, biotin

GAMMALINOLENIC ACID

Helped by zinc and B6

DIHOMO-GAMMALINOLENIC ACID

Helped by vitamin C, vitamin B3
zinc

Arachidonic Acid

PROSTAGLANDINS 1

PROSTAGLANDINS 2

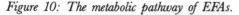

Figure 10: The metabolic pathway of EFAs.

A shortage of any of these 'co-factors' would put a spanner in the works as far as the conversion of EFAs is concerned. In fact, deficiencies of zinc, magnesium or vitamin B6 can actually block the conversion of cis-linoleic acid to gammalinolenic acid.

There have been some studies to show that, in general, people with MS are low in B12, B1, B6, magnesium, zinc, molybdenum and vanadium. The deficiencies may be a result of MS, rather than a cause of them.

In the USA, the late Dr Carl Pfeiffer, who ran the Brain Bio Center in Princeton, New Jersey, found that *all* the MS patients he tested were 'pyroluric' which simply means they were losing zinc and vitamin B6 in the urine. Dr Pfeiffer found that when he made up the deficiency of zinc and B6, plus a supplement of manganese, the patients stabilized. (Pfeiffer's dose was 15mg zinc plus 50mg B6 plus 10mg manganese, twice a day.)

In the UK, doctors specializing in nutritional medicine also give their MS patients zinc plus B6. Sometimes the dose of zinc can be very high indeed. Injections of vitamin B12 are also recommended on a weekly basis, or more frequently.

Free Radicals and Anti-Oxidants

Vitamin C, vitamin E, selenium, and the enzyme super oxide dismutase (S.O.D.) are all anti-oxidants.

It is known that in some circumstances, for example high temperatures, the molecules of essential fatty acids accept oxygen atoms more easily. This is part of the oxidation process. The oxidation process chops fatty acids out of the membranes. These oxygen atoms can then detach themselves and fix into another molecule. These unstable molecules which transport oxygen are called 'free radicals'.

Free radicals can be destructive. There is a loss of integrity of the membranes. All functional controls go by the board and anarchy takes over. So the whole anti-oxidant system is very important.

The B Group of Vitamins

Vitamins B6, B3 (usually called nicotinic acid) and biotin are essential for the biochemical conversion process of essential fatty acids; but the other B vitamins are important too in MS.

Vitamins B1 (Thiamine) and B2 (Riboflavin)

There is some research to show that polyneuritis occurs with B1 deficiencies, and people with MS have been found to be low in B1 and B2. B1 is thought to be effective in improving conditions like neuritis, with numbness of the hands and tingling of the hands and feet. A B2 deficiency can be connected with eye problems (e.g. retrobulbar neuritis, blurred vision), and to nervous symptoms like numbness, tremor, and the inability to pass urine. B2 is crucial in the formation of a number of enzymes. It plays a major role in the metabolism of proteins, fats, and carbohydrates. It enhances the metabolism of vitamin B6, and there is an interrelationship between B2 and B6.

Vitamin B3 (Niacin, Nicotinamide, Nicotinic Acid)

It is thought that people with MS are lacking in this vitamin. B3 forms part of the body's enzyme systems and is essential for the biochemical conversion processes that go on in the body.

Vitamin B6 (pyridoxine)

B6 is necessary for the first stages of the biochemical conversion process of essential fatty acids. B6 seems to play an important role in the health of muscles and nerves

There has been some research to show that patients with MS are deficient in vitamin B6. And the hypothesis has been put forward that a relative B6 deficiency may cause MS in susceptible persons. Exposure to carbon monoxide poisoning increases the need for vitamin B6.

Vitamin B12

Recent research has shown that there are unusual B12 deficiencies in many patients with MS. The reason for this is not clear. It may be because people with MS for some reason have impaired absorption of vitamin B12 from the gastro-intestinal tract.

In any case, as far as MS is concerned, B12 has a role in the maintenance of myelin in the nervous system and it is also needed for folate to be able to work properly.

Some doctors specializing in nutritional medicine give their MS patients an injection of B12 once a week, with reportedly good results. Dr Kingsley says that he has given massive doses of B12 to some patients, starting with injections of 1mg and increasing to 12mg. He reports excellent results in some cases.

Pantothenic Acid

In certain laboratory animals, pantothenic acid deficiency has produced symptoms including the loss of the myelin sheath, and degenerative changes in the spinal cord and peripheral nerves. The need for pantothenic acid is increased under stress, and it is a good anti-stress supplement.

Choline and Inositol

Choline is concerned with the metabolism of fats. It helps in the production of lecithin (phospholipids). Inositol, too, aids in the metabolism of fats and seems to have some effect on muscular tissue.

Folic Acid

Folic acid appears to be concerned with helping new cells to form. It is very important in making blood and in keeping the intestines in good condition. It is also vital in maintaining healthy nerve function. Folic acid may be the commonest vitamin deficiency.

Biotin

Biotin is required by the body to assist in the metabolism of fats. A deficiency of biotin can cause a disturbed nervous system.

Things That Rob You of B Vitamins

The B vitamins are vulnerable to heat, air, and water in cooking. If you cook foods in too much water, the B vitamins will get thrown away with the discarded water down the drain. A lot of B6 and folic acid is destroyed by heat in the cooking process, and some B vitamins get lost when food is exposed to light.

Alcohol, coffee and other drinks containing caffeine have a nasty way of depleting the body of the B vitamins. These stimulants appear to increase the loss of nearly all nutrients which dissolve in water. Research in the USA has shown that caffeine creates a shortage of inositol in the body.

Many of the B vitamins are also made by bacteria in the intestine, but if you are taking an antibiotic this will destroy the bacteria involved in this process.

The B vitamins are synergistic, which means that they work better when they are taken with each other, and with certain other vitamins and minerals (zinc has already been mentioned). Be particularly careful *not* to take B1 on its own.

All the B vitamins must be taken daily, as they are not stored in the body.

Dose

The best way to take the B vitamins is in a commercial 'B complex' tablet.

In addition, you could take one B6 50mg tablet (not more than twice a day) if the dose of B6 in the complex tablet is much lower than this.

Vitamin B6 should always be taken with vitamin B complex.

Vitamin C

Vitamin C is not stored in the body, so it has to be taken daily by dietary means. It has two vital functions connected with MS. It stimulates the formation of prostaglandins made from essential fatty acids. The conversion of dihomo-gammalinolenic acid into prostaglandins 1 is activated by vitamin C, together with zinc and nicotinic acid (B3). The second vital function of vitamin C is as an anti-oxidant. This is vital when you are eating a diet rich in essential fatty acids. Without taking anti-oxidants as well, essential fatty acids could even be dangerous.

Vitamin C is also well known as a detoxifying agent, and as a therapy for infections. It helps the body defend itself against any foreign substance reaching the blood, and increases the bacteria-destroying ability of the white blood cells.

The vitamin C content of foods is destroyed by cooking, both by the heat, and the loss in the water thrown away after cooking, so it is a good idea to take supplements of vitamin C as well as including vitamin C rich foods in your diet, to ensure a high daily intake.

Dose: The ARMS target level for vitamin C is 120mg a day for both men and women. A suitable supplement of vitamin C could contain 1000mg or more twice a day. Vitamin C is non-toxic, and there is no risk in taking high doses.

Vitamin D and Calcium

A hypothesis has been put forward that inadequate supplies of vitamin D and calcium at adolescence, a time of rapid brain growth, may contribute to MS. This is because vitamin D and calcium are needed for normal myelin synthesis and membrane assembly.

Vitamin E

Vitamin E is essential to prevent oxidation of unsaturated fats to dangerous peroxides. It probably also reduces the conversion of essential fatty acids into toxic substances.

Supplements of evening primrose oil or other products containing GLA *must* be taken with vitamin E. Many of the capsules available already contain vitamin E, but some do not.

Red blood cells break down when essential fatty acids which form the cell structure are harmed by oxygen, due to a lack of vitamin E. Muscular weakness can happen if they are not supplied with vitamin E, and the muscles can suffer from an increased content of calcium.

Dose: Supplements of vitamin E could be as high as 600–1000 i.u. per day. The ARMS target is 12mg a day.

Zinc

Zinc is an extremely important trace element, as it forms the composition of at least 160 different enzymes. Indeed, it is the most widely used mineral in the formation of enzymes. These enzymes are involved in digestion, metabolism, and tissue respiration. Zinc is essential for the production of proteins, and the synthesis of DNA – the basis of the genetic code. It also takes a leading role in the processes which ensure normal absorption and function of vitamins, especially the B group.

Zinc is needed in the metabolism of essential fatty acids from which prostaglandins are produced. This means that the immune system cannot work properly without zinc. Each stage of the metabolic pathway of linoleic acid involves zinc. Zinc has an important role to play in the synthesis of PG1. It is also important in maintaining a balance between prostaglandins 1 and prostaglandins 2.

Zinc plays an important role in the specialization of lymphocytes, the white cells. 'T' lymphocytes mature in the thymus (that's why they are called 'T' lymphocytes). These 'T' lymphocytes are the body's army, so they are essential if the immune system is to defend itself properly. Some of these 'T' lymphocytes become T-killers which can destroy their targets; others become T-helpers which can help other white cells make antibodies; and others become T-suppressors which moderate the manufacture of antibodies. The activity of the thymic hormones is also tied up with there being enough zinc.

This vital trace element is mostly found in animal foods. Oysters are the richest source, and meat is a good source. Vegetarians and people who subsist on processed and refined foods may be low in zinc. The cheapest foods tend to be lowest in zinc. There is some evidence too that people who have suffered physical injury or disease increase their excretion of zinc. Alcohol, corticosteroids and the contraceptive pill also cause the loss of zinc from the body.

Zinc teams up with vitamin B6 in the body, particularly for protein synthesis. It seems that our needs for zinc and B6 are increased in what physiologists call situations of helplessness and hopelessness, which means situations in which one has no control.

Dose of zinc: You need to be sure of getting 15mg of *elemental zinc* twice a day. Read the label of supplements containing zinc carefully, as they can be misleading.

(The ARMS target level for zinc in the ARMS diet is only 12mg zinc a day for both men and women.)

Magnesium

A deficiency of magnesium upsets the nerve-muscle functions, and can be associated with tremor, convulsions, over-excitability and behavioural problems. A group of healthy volunteers who went on a diet deficient in magnesium developed muscle spasms and weakness, involuntary twitching and inability to control the bladder. These symptoms all went away when they took magnesium again. Some people with MS in the USA reported that supplements of magnesium got rid of foot cramps.

Magnesium is needed to help linoleic acid convert to gammalinolenic acid – a deficiency of magnesium would get in the way of the conversion process at this step.

Some studies have shown that people with MS are low in magnesium.

Magnesium is closely related to calcium and phosphorus in its metabolic functions. Both calcium outside the cells and magnesium inside the cells are important in helping to transmit nerve impulses to muscles.

Dose: 50mg once a day.

Manganese

Manganese should not be confused with magnesium. The main reason for taking a supplement of manganese is to counterbalance the zinc supplements. This is because as your zinc level goes up, the manganese goes down. For every 15mg of zinc you take, you should at the same time take 10mg manganese.

In animal studies, a deficiency of manganese has been associated with disturbed balance (ataxia), fatigue, depression and allergies. In the experience of Dr Carl Pfeiffer, author of many books about elemental nutrition, all auto-immune diseases respond to manganese.

As a matter of interest, manganese is particularly high in tropical fruits, and spices such as clove, cardamom, ginger, turmeric, cinnamon, black pepper. MS is virtually unknown in those countries where these foods are eaten every day.

Dose: 10mg twice a day.

Selenium

Selenium is a mineral. It is one of the body's protectors, as an anti-oxidant. It is present in an enzyme called glutathione peroxidase (GTP). The various substances which attack cells are rapidly destroyed by GTP before they can cause any damage. Lack of selenium reduces the efficiency of GTP, and body cells are then open to danger. The white blood cells also contain high amounts of GTP. As an anti-oxidant, selenium should be taken together with vitamin C and vitamin E.

People with MS are believed to be low in selenium.

The functions of selenium include: maintenance of the immune system through the white blood cells; protection against toxic materials such as cadmium and mercury; the production of prostaglandins; an anti-inflammatory effect; protection against free radicals; a synergistic action with vitamin E in maintaining the functions of mitochondria, the energy-producing apparatus in all body cells.

The recommended dietary intake is not exceeding 200mg a day.

Dose: 50µg twice a day.

Vanadium

Vanadium is a trace element. A study done at Reading University in 1984 by Dr Neil Ward and Professor Derek Bryce-Smith and others showed that patients with MS had low levels of vanadium.

Deficiency states in animals show up in reduction in red blood cell production; increased blood fat level; and increased blood cholesterol levels. It has functions in fat metabolism and blood production.

Daily intakes of vanadium in the diet are probably between 100 and 300mg. Best food sources are parsley, radishes, lettuce, strawberries, calf's liver, sardines, cucumber and apples.

Lecithin

Lecithin plays a vital role in the metabolism of fats. In her book *Let's Get Well*, Adelle Davis says that autopsy studies on MS people showed a marked decrease in the lecithin content of the brain and myelin sheath covering the nerves, both of which are normally high in lecithin. The lecithin in people with MS is also, apparently, abnormal, containing saturated instead of unsaturated fats.

Lecithin is continuously produced by the liver, passes into the intestine with bile and is absorbed into the blood. It aids in the transportation of fats, helps the cells remove fats and cholesterol from the blood, and serves as a structural material for every cell in the body, particularly in the brain and nerves.

Lecithin consists of several substances which require essential fatty acids, choline, and inositol for their structure, and numerous other nutrients to synthesize them. If these other raw materials are in short supply, lecithin is not manufactured efficiently in the body. These other nutrients include vitamin B6 and magnesium.

Dose: 2 tablets of 200mg, three times a day.

The Healing Waters of Gornja Trepca

There is one spa in what was formerly Yugoslavia which has earned the reputation of being very beneficial to MS sufferers. Some scientists have analysed the spring water and found that it does have special properties and that it contains elements rarely found in spring water. Gornja Trepca has acquired the name of 'atomic spa' because it has increased radioactivity. The spring contains such micro-elements as cesium, rubidium, strontium, radium, and also lithium, cobalt, vanadium, titanium, uranium, radon, manganese and other constituents. The most unusual element is cesium. It is found here in a concentration very rare in European water. The spa is recommended in the treatment of MS by the authorities there.

Amino Acids

Until now the emphasis with nutritional supplements has been on vitamins, minerals, and essential fatty acids. But one essential metabolite has been missing from this team – amino acids.

Amino acids are the building blocks of proteins. All tissue in the body is made from amino acids – every cell, every muscle, each hair and nail, all of the 15,000 enzymes and each chemical in the brain is made from amino acids. They are crucial to the biochemistry of the body. The highly complex molecular logic of our bodies, with its intricate metabolic pathways, needs the right nutrients in the right amount to function smoothly and efficiently. These nutrients are vitamins, minerals, fatty acids *and* amino acids and other metabolites derived from them, all working synergistically in harmony.

Amino acids are as important as any of these other nutrients, and a lack of any of them can have a cascade of consequences on health and well-being. The philosophy of doctors specializing in nutritional medicine is that every disorder is the result of metabolic imbalances, rather than a single specific cause. They believe that, just as imbalances can cause disorders, so correcting the metabolic imbalances can put right disorders. Until very recently, amino acids were left out of this equation.

We have already seen what can happen to the body if it is lacking in essential fatty acids, vitamins and minerals. If the body lacks amino acids, it simply degenerates.

There are 22 amino acids, capable of producing over 50,000 different protein structures. Eight of these are called essential amino acids because the body cannot make them itself so you have to eat the protein foods to get them. These eight are called phenylalanine, tryptophan, methionine, lysine, leucine, isoleucine, valine and threonine.

From these eight amino acids, the body can use metabolic pathways to synthesize all the others. The non-essential amino acids include tyrosine, asparagine, ornithine, histidine, glutamic acid, glutamine, proline and glycine.

Without amino acids, human life would not exist. They supply the raw materials for maintaining the genetic code – DNA – as well as for repairing damaged tissue, for cell division, for making enzymes, for building new connective tissue and for making hormones which regulate bodily processes and neurotransmitters.

It makes sense to take amino acids for multiple sclerosis, a degenerative disease in which you need all the help you can get to repair damaged tissue.

Amino acids are not drugs, and are not toxic. They are like the broken-down molecules of food. They cannot do you any harm, and they might well do you some good. People with MS who have taken 'free-form' amino acids report an immediate boost in energy and an end to that draining symptom of MS, fatigue.

Why You Should Take Amino Acid Supplements

If you are eating a good healthy diet with lots of protein, such as meat, fish and eggs, you may wonder why you should be taking amino acid supplements at all. The answer is that your body may not be processing the protein you are eating properly. Faulty protein digestion can result in partial amino acid deficiency, even if you are eating a lot of protein in your daily diet. If you are suffering from fatigue, and if your body is showing some signs of degeneration, then the protein you are eating may not be reaching the places it is most needed.

One possible cause of this is not chewing your food properly. Other possible causes are factors which can decrease the output of digestive chemicals, such as emotional stress, eating junk food, not enough exercise, viruses, pollution, injury, drugs (e.g. cannabis), and genetic disorders.

Children are usually told to chew their food properly, and there are sound reasons for this. Chewing properly tears the food apart, breaks it down, and helps to release digestive substances. The more thoroughly you chew, the more nutrients your body will absorb. But if you gobble your food and bolt it down, the acids and enzymes don't have as large a surface area of food to work on, so when the food reaches the gut, less of it is digested. As a result, fewer amino acids are absorbed into the body to carry out the vital protein synthesis.

Once this happens you are caught in a vicious circle, because one of the important roles of protein synthesis is to manufacture digestive enzymes. If there is poor protein synthesis, there will be fewer enzymes to digest the food, and fewer amino acids will be released from the food to build the body's tissues.

The knock-on effect from this can be quite dramatic, as amino acids have such varied and vital functions. As the number of amino acids drops, it has an effect on hormone production, with less insulin to regulate blood sugar levels, less adrenalin to help you cope with stress, less thyroxin to carry out body metabolism and less thymosin to stimulate the immune system.

Body tissues show the signs of a shortage of amino acids – muscle tone will fade, skin will slacken, nails will become soft and split.

A shortage of amino acids can greatly affect your mood and well-being. You are likely to get tired easily and to suffer from bouts of anxiety and depression. You are more susceptible to disease, and you may show signs of premature ageing.

How To Take Amino Acids

The best way to take amino acids is to take supplements of free-form amino acids, either in powder form or capsules. Free-form amino acids are amino acids which have been separated in the laboratory from their parent molecules. Free-form amino acids require no digestion whatsoever. They are taken straight through the gut walls and into the bloodstream. Free-form amino acid treatment is very fast; some people report feeling the effects of them virtually straight away. The most likely effects with MS are a boost in energy levels, a lessening of fatigue, and the disappearance of hypoglycaemia.

Free-form amino acids can help particularly against allergies and auto-immune diseases, of which multiple sclerosis can be counted as one. They work by strengthening the natural metabolic reactions in the body, with the help of vitamin and mineral co-factors (especially vitamins B3, B6, and C). Some doctors who have been using free-form amino acids in the treatment of multiple sclerosis include all the sulphur-based amino acids because these work by improving the state of body tissue. These amino acids are methionine, taurine, cysteine and cystine.

Methionine also works as a way of helping to rid the body of mercury and other heavy metals (lead, cadmium) toxicity, as it is a chelator, latching on to the toxic metals and escorting them out of the body.

You can buy free-form amino acids yourself in a health food shop or by mail order and treat yourself, but it is better to consult a nutritionally oriented doctor, if possible. S/he will be able to give you some specific tests to find out your amino acid profile, so s/he can come up with a prescription which is tailor-made to your specific needs. There is a particular test known as the urinary amino test which can analyse the amino acids in your urine, and identify any deficits.

Ideally, free-form amino acids should be taken on an empty stomach twice a day, first thing in the morning and last thing at night, or as directed by your doctor. If you are taking the powdered form, dissolve half a teaspoon in half a tumbler of water, washed down with another half tumbler of water. Always take amino acids with the vitamin and mineral co-factors, as described earlier in this chapter.

As well as boosting your energy levels, free-form amino acids should also have the effect of reducing the sensation of feeling weak with hunger, the hypoglycaemia common in MS caused by low blood sugar levels. This is because the hormone insulin regulates blood sugar levels and insulin production is dependent upon amino acids.

The following clinics use nutritional and environmental medicine to treat MS:

Dr Patrick Kingsley
72 Main Street
Osgathorpe
Leics LE12 9TA
Tel: 01530 223622

The Hale Clinic
7 Park Crescent
London W1N 3HE
Tel: 0171-631 0156

The Castle Street Clinic
36 Castle Street
Guildford
Surrey GU1 3UQ
Tel: 01425 461740

Biolab Medical Unit
The Stone House
9 Weymouth Street
London W1N 3FF
Tel: 0171-636 5959

The Centre for the Study of
  Complementary Medicine
51 Bedford Place
Southampton
Hampshire SO15 2DT
Tel: 01703 334752

and:

14 Harley House
Upper Harley Street
London NW1 4PR
Tel: 0171-935 7848

A private hospital specialising in nutritional medicine is:

Breakspear Hospital
Belswains Lane
Hemel Hempstead
Herts HP3 9HP
Tel: 0144 261333

See also Chapter 9.

Lactobacillus acidophilus (or similar products)

The gut is populated with two predominant groups of bacteria, the putrefactive *Bacteroides* and the beneficial *Bifidobacteria*. The aim of taking supplements such as *Lactobacillus acidophilus*, probion, or similar products, is to promote the correct balance between the two main types of bacteria.

Degenerative conditions, like multiple sclerosis, are believed by some practitioners to be connected with an imbalance of the putrefactive *Bacteroides* against the healthier *Bifidobacteria*, with a consequent build-up of toxicity in the system. A disease such as MS indicates that the inner environment of the body is unbalanced, with a depletion of oxygen and essential nutrients, and auto-intoxication.

Taking supplements of acidophilus will help re-establish healthy intestinal flora.

One of the big advantages of taking acidophilus or a similar product is that it will help bring about regular and easy bowel movements (see section on constipation, page 225). Taking acidophilus will also help bring Candida albicans under control.

Dose: One 500mg acidophilus capsule 1-3 times a day. (Or if taking a similar product, follow the directions on the tub.)

CONCLUSION

Here is a complete list of supplements beneficial to people with MS, together with their suggested doses.

- Evening primrose oil capsules: ideally, 9 capsules a day. 3 capsules of 500mg, three times a day with meals.
- Fish oil capsules: 1000mg fish lipid, one capsule a day. Or combine evening primrose oil with fish oil in one capsule.
- Vitamin C: Up to 1 gram per tablet. One three times a day.
- Vitamin E: Up to 1000 iu per tablet. One three times a day.
- B complex (all the B vitamins in balance): Any commercial product should supply adequate amounts in the right ratios. 1 three times a day.
- B6: 50mg once or twice a day (no more).
- B12: Injections once a week or more often. 1mg (or more) hydroxycobalamin.
- Zinc: 15mg at least elemental zinc twice a day.
- Manganese: 10 mg twice a day.
- Selenium: 50 µg twice a day.
- Molybdenum: Trace amounts.
- Lecithin: 2 tablets of 200mg, three times a day.
- Free-form amino acids: ½ teaspoon in water twice a day.
- Acidophilus (or similar product): Up to three doses of 500mg a day.

It is possible to find vitamin, mineral and trace element products which combine some of these nutrients in one tablet, which saves the bother of having to take several different supplements.[1]

All these fatty acids, vitamins, minerals, trace elements and amino acids work together as a team, so it is important to take them in the right balance, and not take huge amounts of certain nutrients and nothing of other ones.

The above doses are approximations. If you can see a nutritionally qualified practitioner who can give you an accurate nutritional profile, then supplements and doses can be tailor-made to your particular needs.

1. The one I take is called 'Lamberts Health Insurance Plus'. Available from:

Lamberts Healthcare Ltd
1 Lamberts Road
Tunbridge Wells
Kent TN2 3EQ
Tel: 01892 552120

9

Food Allergies and Environmental Medicine

In recent years, the whole subject of food allergies has gained in popularity and even in an acceptance by some doctors. This whole area is sometimes called environmental medicine, or clinical ecology.

ENVIRONMENTAL MEDICINE

Environmental medicine is the study of how the environment promotes disease or ill health in individuals. The most common environmental factors which can bring about ill health are foods and chemicals. The aim of an environmental medicine practitioner is to use various techniques to pinpoint the foods, chemicals or other substances which might be causing the problem, to exclude those toxic substances from the patient's lifestyle, and to detoxify the body. This has to be done on an individual basis, as one substance can be perfectly benign to one person yet toxic to another.

THE DEFINITION OF 'ALLERGY'

There may be many doctors who take issue with the word 'allergy' being used in the way I am using it in this book.

Most immunologists take the view that 'allergy' only involves those reactions in which a specific immunologic (antigen-antibody) reaction can be demonstrated. This is the narrow definition of the word 'allergy'.

A wider definition of 'allergy' includes supersensitivity to substances which have no known immunologic basis. This more generalized term is in keeping with the word 'allergy' originally coined by the Austrian physician Clemens von Pirquet at the beginning of this century. Von Pirquet himself stated that the term 'allergy' involved the general concept of changed reactivity.

This wider definition of 'allergy' which does not necessarily involve antigen-antibody reactions, is in current usage today. It is in this broad sense that the term 'allergy' is used in this book.

FOOD ALLERGIES

Testing for food allergies is one part of the job of a practitioner in environmental and nutritional medicine. Another part is to test for other things that could be toxic to the individual, such as mercury in your dental fillings, cigarette smoke, or chemicals such as pesticides, for example.

Over the last 15 years or so there have been some very well-documented individual successes of people with MS who have excluded certain foods from their diet, and their MS has improved – sometimes dramatically – as a result.

Everything in this chapter is based on 'anecdotal evidence' – a number of individual case histories added together. We are now in the field of 'alternative medicine' where practitioners take issue with the conventional scientific method and the approach of suppressing symptoms. As each MS person may be allergic to a different set of foods and substances, it would be impossible to set up an orthodox controlled trial. However, many of the practitioners of environmental and nutritional medicine are doctors trained in orthodox medicine, but who have gone over to the other camp because they have become disillusioned with various aspects of orthodox medicine.

The main MS groups in the UK, the MS Society and ARMS, both dismiss the field of environmental medicine as being unproven and unscientific. I think it is a pity they both take this attitude. I personally have met several people who swear by the food allergy approach, and whose lives have improved immeasurably as a result of excluding the foods and substances to which they were sensitive. So, if you want hard proof, you won't find it here. But I think it is wise to be open-minded on this topic, as hard proof is never likely to be forthcoming in this realm.

Dr Patrick Kingsley, one of the leading doctors practising environmental and nutritional medicine in the UK, has treated hundreds of MS patients in this way. At a conservative estimate he claims that more than 50 per cent of these MS patients have improved as a result of excluding the foods and substances to which they were found to be reacting. In other words, they have got better, rather than got worse. As well as excluding allergic foods, doctors practising environmental and nutritional medicine prescribe a wide range of nutritional supplements for their MS patients (see previous chapter).

Test Yourself for Food Allergies Before Starting Any Diet for MS

If the food allergists are right, you should test yourself for your particular food allergies *before* starting on the ARMS Essential Fatty Acid Diet, or the Swank Low-Fat Diet or any other diet suggested for MS. If you are allergic to milk, for example, you should not eat *any* milk products, no matter how skimmed or low-fat they may be.

You might find you are allergic to perfectly 'healthy' foods which are recommended on the ARMS diet, such as tomatoes, or green peppers, apples, or bananas, for example.

To find out which foods you are allergic to would take two to three visits to one of the practitioners of environmental medicine. This would be fairly expensive, but there is not much point saving £100–£150 if the foods you eat are making you worse.

Anyone interested in the environmental medicine approach to MS should contact:

British Society for Allergy, Environmental and
    Nutritional Medicine
PO Box 28
Totton
Southampton SO40 2ZA
Tel: 01703 812124

See Useful Addresses for more clinics using nutritional and environmental medicine to treat MS.

Food Allergies and MS

When the body's immune system has gone wrong, as with MS, you can show abnormal reactions to foods which a normal healthy person could eat without any bad effects.

Allergy symptoms include: tiredness after meals, palpitations, headache, nausea, bloating, high pulse rate and sweating. In MS, these can also include cold legs, constricted breathing, difficulties with vision, lethargy, depression and a rapid onset of MS symptoms.

Are Food Allergies the Cause of MS, or the Result of Having MS?

It is not clear whether food and other allergies are the *result* of having MS, or in some way involved in *causing* the disease.

For a long time naturopaths have believed that toxic substances cause chronic illness. At long last, some conventionally-trained doctors are catching up with the naturopaths and looking scientifically at how food and other substances can be toxic to an individual.

The offending food may give you a specific symptom. It could be, for example, that cane sugar makes your eyes go hazy, or that grapefruit juice makes your speech more slurred.

Thanks to the work of Dr Richard Mackarness who wrote *Not All In The Mind* (Pan), we know that the foods you crave most and eat most habitually are likely to be the very foods you are allergic to. This is unfortunate, but true. In his book *Chemical Victims* Dr Mackarness also made people aware of 'masked allergies'. Roughly, this means you are addicted to various foods and substances, and you get symptoms when you *don't* have them – rather like withdrawal symptoms from a drug.

Orthodox doctors tend to dismiss the possibility of food allergies, saying that, once eaten, all foods get broken down in the digestive process to the same basic molecules anyway, so it shouldn't make any difference what you eat. These doctors also tend to take umbrage at the misuse of the word 'allergy'.

But doctors who specialize in environmental and nutritional

medicine are convinced there is a link between eating food to which you may be sensitive, and a whole range of different symptoms.

Some neurologists have also had to join the food allergy camp when they have seen the evidence with their own eyes. One such is the American neurologist, Dr Robert Soll, who now runs a clinic in Iowa where he treats MS patients using allergy techniques.

Dr Soll evolved the idea that 'individuals with multiple sclerosis frequently display a profile of numerous allergies . . . This condition might . . . cause the absorption of endotoxin from the intestines and an attack of MS'.

Dr Soll's definition of endotoxins is the release of bacterial poisons, produced by an infection. In his book *MS: Something Can Be Done and You Can Do It* (Contemporary Books) he says:

The intestinal tract may represent a large reservoir of endotoxin, and very small quantities of the substance may be absorbed through a weakened, inflamed intestinal wall as would result from the ingestion of allergic foods. Thus, an infection, which would cause a greater release of endotoxin into the bloodstream, not only causes fever and cold hands and cold feet, but also an acute exacerbation of MS. On the other hand, inflammation of the bowel wall resulting in absorption of endotoxin could produce a slow, cumulative adverse effect day after day, contributing to the slow, downhill course we see so often in MS patients.

In his book Dr Soll quotes several cases of people with MS, who have very dramatic 'before and after' stories. In each case, he isolated the foods to which these people were allergic, and the foods were banned. These patients were also treated with antibiotics each time they had an infection.

Possible Mechanisms For Certain Foods Causing Allergies

The mechanism for certain foods causing allergies in some MS people probably involves the gut. Semi-digested food is getting through permeable intestine walls. Perhaps this permeability is caused by a profileration of candida (see page 122).

Damage to the intestinal mucosa

A possible reason why the intestinal mucosa is damaged may be because of a cow's milk allergy which began very early in the person's life, perhaps even as early as the first days.

In western societies, the period around birth is disturbed dramatically. Ideally, the baby should be able to suck at its mother's breast within the first hour or so after the birth. The baby's first food is colostrum. Colostrum contains special antibodies (IgA) able to protect the intestinal mucosa.

However, few babies get the optimum amount of colostrum in their first days of life. Many babies born in hospital – even those whose mothers want to breastfeed – are given a small bottle of formula, and so, in effect, they are given foreign proteins, to which the baby may become sensitive for the rest of his life.

Malabsorption

If there is damage to the lining of the gastro-intestinal tract, and food is seeping through the gut walls, it also means that the food you eat is not being absorbed properly. If malabsorption is a problem, then the body will be deficient in minerals, vitamins, and trace elements. This in itself would have a fairly catastrophic cascade of consequences.

Too much tea or coffee can also block the absorption of all the minerals, and some vitamins.

Abnormal Immune Reactions

The immune system seems to be involved in the mechanism of food allergies too. In a complex way which is not fully understood, the immune system decides that these food substances are foreign bodies, and sets the troops in motion against body tissues. It is thought that the immunoglobulins are involved in this. These are large protein molecules manufactured by special white cells, the B lymphocytes.

Immunoglobulins are proteins and their detailed chemical structure is designed to bind specifically to the chemicals or bacteria defined as foreign, i.e. non-self. Under normal circumstances the body is able to recognize itself and so does not make immunoglobulins (or antibodies) which destroy its own structures.

Recent research shows that there is an abnormality of immunoglobulins in 54.5 per cent of MS patients. No one has yet made any link between this fact and the possibility of food allergies.

Proliferation of Candida and Leaky Mucous Membranes

There is evidence that there is a connection between yeast and MS. No one is saying that candida is the cause of MS, merely that there is a connection, and that once the candida is treated the patient's condition will improve.

Candida albicans is a yeast-like organism, commonly known as thrush. Candida albicans figures prominently in the intestinal tract of humans. Under normal circumstances, candida albicans is an innocent bystander. But the trouble starts when the candida changes from its normal yeast-like form, to a mycelial fungal form. The yeast-like state is nothing to worry about. But the fungal form produces long root-like mycelia which can penetrate the mucous membrane of the intestine. This penetration can lead to leaky mucous membranes in the digestive tract. This allows incompletely digested substances (e.g. proteins from the diet) to come into direct contact with the immune system. This is why people with a chronic overgrowth of candida albicans often have many food and other allergies.

As well as causing a leaky intestinal mucous membrane, candida also produces a specific toxin called candida toxin. This can weaken the entire immune system, and make it less able to deal with allergy problems. (See page 122 for more on candida.)

The Commonest Foods to which People with MS are Allergic

The commonest foods to which people with MS are allergic are:

Milk and all dairy produce
Yeast (in bread etc.)
All fungi (mushrooms etc.) and fermented products (e.g. vinegar)
Sugar
Potatoes
Tea and anything with tannin

Dr Patrick Kingsley, who has had more experience in this field than any other doctor in the UK, finds that wheat, barley, oats and rye (the gluten grains, see page 133) are not common foods for MS people to be allergic to. However, some of the foods made with these grains do contain *yeast*, and this could be the problem. He also finds that chemicals do not feature very prominently with MS people, although mercury in dental fillings is common (see chapter 11). Interestingly, Dr Kingsley is convinced that mercury and other toxic metals are the underlying cause of MS. Second to this come food intolerances. Next, a deficiency in vitamin B12 (which he gives in megadoses), vitamin B1, and magnesium.

Other doctors however, both in the UK and in the USA, would also include wheat, red meat, fruits and some vegetables in their top ten list of foods to which MS people are most commonly allergic.

Remember that different foods affect different people differently. Even so, be very suspicious of milk, all dairy produce, all sugars, yeast and all fungi (e.g. mushrooms), fruit, wheat, red meat, tea, vegetables.

If you change your attitude to the culprit foods and think of them as poisons, it's not so hard to give them up completely. If you identify chemical pollutants, the same thing applies. Change your lifestyle so you avoid them completely.

What To Avoid On A Cow's Milk-Free Diet

- Cow's milk (even in very small quantities)
- Creamed foods
- Creamed sauces
- Fresh cream
- Cow's milk cheeses of every description
- Cow's milk yogurt
- Custard
- Milk chocolate and some dark chocolate
- Butter
- Dairy ice cream
- Condensed milk
- Dried evaporated milk
- Powdered milk
- Malted milk
- Ovaltine

- Drinking chocolate
- Manufactured salad dressings
- Batter
- Soups with added milk
- Most margarines, because they contain whey (only a very few do not)
- Foods fried in butter
- Cakes, biscuits and bread with milk in them
- Any packaged foods containing milk powder, lactose, whey or casein.

If your symptoms improve on a cow's milk free diet, you can introduce either goat's milk or its products (e.g. cheese and yogurt) *or* soya milk, but not both at the same time. Ewe's milk can also be tried.

Remember – read labels!

What To Avoid on a Yeast-Free and Sugar-Free Diet

- Foods that contain yeast as an ingredient: biscuits, breads, pastries, cakes and cake mixes, flour enriched with vitamins from yeast, and meat fried in crumbs.
- The following contain yeast or yeast-like substances because of their nature or the nature of their manufacture and preparation: mushrooms, cheeses, vinegar such as apple, pear, cider, grape and malt vinegars (although some vinegar is pure chemical acetic acid which could be allowed if you could find some and be sure about it). These vinegars should be avoided in their original state as well as in such foods as mayonnaise, olives, pickles, sauerkraut, horseradish, french dressing and tomato sauce. Also avoid stock cubes, yeast extracts and gravy mixes.
- Fermented drinks: whisky, gin, wine, brandy, rum, vodka, beer, in fact *all* alcoholic drinks.
- Malted products: cereals, most chocolate and malted milk drinks.
- Citrus fruit juices, either frozen or canned, melons. Only home-squeezed fruit juices are yeast-free.
- Many vitamin products are derived from yeast, or have their sources from yeast.

- Because yeasts feed on sugar and carbohydrate, sugar in all forms *must* be avoided: white and brown sugar, honey, maple syrup, golden syrup, sweets, toffees, chocolates, candies, ice cream, biscuits, puddings, drinks with added sugar such as squashes, Britvic orange and lemon juice, Coca Cola, Pepsi Cola and virtually all pop and fizzy drinks including bitter lemon and tonic water.
- White flour in all forms (such as bread, biscuits, puddings, pasta, cakes) etc. which is so heavily refined that yeasts treat it like sugar.

As so many people crave sugar, when you start on a sugar-free diet avoid all sugar substitutes such as saccharine, Saxine, Sweetex, Candarel and so on, or you will never lose your sweet tooth.

What To Avoid on a Tannin-Free Diet

- Tea, Indian and China
- Dark-skinned grapes and plums
- Their dried fruits: e.g. currants, raisins and prunes
- All drinks made from the above fruits, e.g. dark sherry, brandy, red wine, and non-alcoholic drinks from the dark grape.

You may have sultanas (golden raisins), herbal teas that are tannin-free (check the labels) and fruit juices that are yeast- and sugar-free.

What To Avoid on a Totally Caffeine-Free Diet

- Coffee of all sorts, pure ground, bagged, percolated and instant
- Nearly all decaffeinated coffees contain a little caffeine, so avoid them as well
- Chocolate, cocoa, chocolate drinks
- Coca-Cola and all cola drinks
- Coffee-coated cakes
- Some painkillers contain caffeine, so check labels

It is probably *not* wise to drink chicory or similar 'coffee substitutes' instead so avoid them.

MS, Sinusitis and Milk Allergy

In early 1986, there was a flurry of interest about the connection between MS and sinusitis. A paper, plus correspondence on the subject, was published in *The Lancet*.

The doctors (Professor George Dick and Dr Derek Gray) found that in a study of 135 patients with MS, covering 16 GP practices, 65.9 per cent of them had histories of sinusitis on their medical records.

They found that naso-pharyngeal infections, and chronic sinusitis were seventeen times more common in the MS patients than in the controls. These figures do strongly suggest that there is an association between sinusitis and MS.

The doctors conducting this study observed that the peak of sinusitis happened one year before the first attack of MS.

Professor Dick and Dr Gray believe that sinusitis and MS may be causally associated, since sinusitis and sino-mucosal damage precede MS. They also note that sinusitis is common in children aged 5-10. Whatever it is that causes MS is supposed to happen in the first 15 years of life.

A naturopath or a practitioner of environmental and nutritional medicine faced with a patient with sinusitis would immediately suspect a milk allergy. According to Dr Patrick Kingsley, 'Sinusitis is a clear indication of a milk allergy.'

It is very sad that conventionally-trained doctors regard suggestions such as this as rubbish. But I think it is foolish to dismiss out of hand such startling correlations – that most people with MS suffer from milk allergy, and that 65 per cent of MS people get chronic recurrent sinusitis.

Surely it would be sensible to test anyone with MS who gets chronic sinusitis for milk allergy as the next step in the investigations? Removing milk and milk products from these patients might have benefits both for their sinusitis and also their MS.

Early weaning is another factor which can explain the frequency of cow's milk allergy in our society. Babies are fed cow's milk before their digestive system is ready for anything except their mother's milk. This early allergy to cow's milk has long-term consequences and paves the way for allergies later in life.

Of all the foods to which MS people are allergic, cow's milk is top of the list.

Sugar and MS

Another food in the 'Top Ten' list of allergic foods to people with MS is sugar. If someone takes 100 grams of sugar in the form of glucose, fructose, sucrose, honey, or even orange juice, there is a significant drop in the efficiency of white blood cells defending the body. The body's defence system reaches peak weakness two hours after eating any of these foods.

These particular white blood cells, called neutrophyl phagocytes, form around 60-70 per cent of the total white blood cells. This effect leaves the body open to invaders. The more sugar given, the more the immune system is inhibited. It is thought that the effect is the result of increased insulin activity which competes with vitamin C for transport binding sites in the body.

Hypoglycaemia

A symptom not usually associated with multiple sclerosis is hypoglycaemia – low blood sugar. The person may feel light-headed and weak, and crave something sweet.

The worst thing you can do to alleviate hypoglycaemia is to eat something sweet, such as sweets or biscuits. This simply sets you up to repeat the pattern endlessly. If you do eat foods such as these, your blood sugar will shoot up temporarily, but it will quickly drop down to a low level again leaving you hypoglycaemic, weak, and craving something sweet.

Fluctuating blood sugar levels are a sure sign that there is something wrong nutritionally which needs to be sorted out, with a correct diet plus vitamin and mineral supplements.

Instead of going for sugar-laden foods, eat complex carbohydrates, like potatoes in their jackets or wholewheat pasta, which will give a much slower-release type of sugar and help keep your blood sugar levels more stable.

Once you stop eating sugar altogether, cut out all junk foods, switch to a healthy nutritious diet, and take supplements, hypoglycaemia as a symptom should disappear completely.

Candida and MS

Intestinal candidiasis is a major cause of food allergy. Once this is treated, patients complaining of food allergies often improve.

The link between candida and MS has been written about by an American doctor, William G Crook MD in his book *The Yeast Connection* (published by Professional Books). It was another American, Dr Orion Truss, who was the first ecologist to recognize the problem of candida.

In *The Yeast Connection* Dr Crook mentions several cases of patients with MS who, from their medical history, seemed good candidates for anti-candida treatment. In all the cases described in his book, the MS symptoms improved as the candida was treated.

The following case history comes from the book *Nutritional Medicine* by Dr Stephen Davies and Dr Alan Stewart (Pan Books Ltd, 1987). It illustrates how successful a nutritional approach to multiple sclerosis can be.

'Susan was a 29-year-old mother of two who had developed blurred vision, pins and needles, loss of balance, and weakness in the legs and one hand. She had been diagnosed as having multiple sclerosis. Full history-taking revealed that she almost certainly had chronic yeast (candida) problems. Nutritional assessment showed multiple nutrient deficiencies, despite a sensible 'well-balanced' diet, suggesting a problem with absorption of nutrients. She also had telltale signs of food allergy (gut symptoms, eczema in childhood, migraine). Treating her for chronic candidiasis, treating her for food allergies, and correcting her nutritional deficiencies, including vitamin B12 injections (as she was found to be functionally deficient in it) resulted in a marked improvement, to the point that she became symptom-free within a month of commencing treatment. Whilst spontaneous remissions are quite common in multiple sclerosis, this case is probably a demonstration of how, after removing certain 'loads' (deficiencies, candida, food allergy), the body is better able to heal itself. One and a half years later Susan is still symptom-free, with no evidence of any recurrence according to her six-monthly check-ups with a neurologist. Furthermore, she feels fitter than at any time during her adult life.'

What Can Make Someone Sensitive to Candida?

Antibiotics

The story can usually be traced to the patient's childhood, when there may have been recurrent infections – such as urinary tract infections or sinusitis – which have been treated with antibiotics. Antibiotics are very non-selective about which bacteria they kill – they destroy all of them, both good and bad. This upsets the delicate balance of bacteria.

The Contraceptive Pill

The artificial hormones in contraceptive pills mess about with many processes in the body. The known metabolic abnormalities produced by the pill include zinc deficiency, too much copper, altered liver function, changes in many hormonal levels, and gross changes in the function of many enzymes. Many women with MS who also have candida also take the pill.

The pill alters and depresses the immune system and changes the acidity of vaginal secretions. This often results in thrush.

Sulphonamide Drugs

These drugs are prescribed for conditions such as cystitis (a urinary tract infection). Again, patients who have MS and who have candida sensitivity are frequently found to have taken sulphonamide drugs.

Steroid Drugs

Candida is more likely in patients who have been receiving large doses of steroids. It is quite common for patients with MS to be given oral steroids when they have an attack of MS. The contraceptive pill is also a steroid drug.

It is not uncommon for someone with MS, especially females, to have been treated with antibiotics and sulphonamide drugs, and been on the contraceptive pill, in the years prior to diagnosis of MS.

The Signs and Symptoms of Chronic Candidiasis

The most common sign of candida is thrush. Thrush is an acute infection, or overgrowth of candida. In children, it can occur in the mouth and gastro-intestinal tract. In adult males it can show up as a sore penis; in females it is a sore vagina, with a white discharge. Thrush can result after a course of antibiotics.

With chronic candidiasis, the symptoms are almost endless. They range from vaginal irritation, to malaise, to headache.

Once the body has chronic candidiasis, it is unbalanced and predisposed to a variety of ecological problems, including food allergies and other sensitivities.

People who already have something wrong with their immune systems are more open to candidiasis. The irony is that they are doubly at risk if they are also taking immunosuppressive drugs.

At a recent symposium on candidiasis, an American physician, Dr Jack Remington, said: 'When we use corticosteroids, antibiotics and cytotoxic drugs in such quantities, we are adding insult to injury. We have to use these drugs, of course, but they cause as much immunosuppression as the underlying disease.'

Treatment

You can find out whether you are sensitive to candida by the same techniques as are used to detect food allergies.

Candida, like all forms of yeast, loves sugar and moist places. The most common treatment is to exclude from your diet: all yeast, all sugars, white flour, cakes, biscuits, coffee, alcohol, tea, mushrooms, cheese. Also, do not eat anything mouldy.

An anti-fungal drug called Nystatin[1] is sometimes prescribed. Doctors who specialize in nutritional medicine would probably also recommend vitamin and mineral supplements, plus evening primrose oil.

Acidophilus is sometimes prescribed to restore the bacteria in the gut to the right balance. Acidophilus is a friendly bacteria found in such foods as live yogurt. However, if you were allergic to milk products you could not take live yogurt. Acidophilus is available in tablet or powder form.

1. Note: Dr Stephen Davies, co-author of *Nutritional Medicine* has a note of caution about Nystatin. He says: 'In some situations, anti-candida treatment with Nystatin can cause an acute exacerbation of the condition, so one should progress very cautiously in MS.'

TESTING YOURSELF FOR FOOD ALLERGIES

If you think you may be allergic to any foods or chemicals, the first thing to do is to get yourself tested for this.

In the last few years, tests for food allergies have progressed by leaps and bounds. Until very recently, the only way to find out to which foods you were allergic was to go through the laborious process of going on a cleansing fast, and then trying each food one by one. This is still an effective self-help method, and cheaper than the other alternatives, but it does take quite a long time, and is better done under supervision.

The Do-It-Yourself Approach

The principle behind testing for food allergies is that you can only find out to which foods you are allergic if you go on a strict cleansing fast first to clear out impurities from the body. Some doctors recommend a complete fast, but others reckon it is safe to start with a cleansing diet of low-risk foods.

The Cleansing Diet – Eating Only Low-Risk Foods

For five to seven days, go on a cleansing fast eating only low-risk foods.

The low-risk foods, to which very few people are allergic, are: lamb, pears, cod, trout, plaice, carrots, courgettes, avocado pears, runner beans, parsnips, swedes, turnips.

For these 5-7 days, these foods can be eaten in any quantity.

While you are casting off toxins into the bloodstream, you will probably not feel very well. That will have passed by the fifth day. On the sixth day, you should feel well enough to start testing the foods.

Testing the Foods, One by One

At the end of the 5-7 days, you can begin testing other foods, one by one. This is not as arduous as it sounds. Once you have passed a food as safe, you can carry on eating it, together with your new food. So you could be eating large and varied meals within a matter of days. There is no limit on quantity.

Begin with foods which many people find 'safe' i.e. they do not react to them. This list includes broccoli, beef, rice, melon, pineapple, lettuce, apples, grapes, and chicken.

Introduce these one per meal. Separate the meals by 5-6 hours. Look out for a reaction, which can normally be expected to happen in this space of time. Allow 2 days to test wheat, corn, oats, and rye as they can have a delayed reaction.

Foods from the same food family should be spaced out. They should not be introduced within 4 days of each other.

By testing new foods one at a time, you can easily see if that food gives you any symptoms. If you get no reaction, you can add that food to the next meal. For example, if you had tested lamb safely, and rice safely, you could eat lamb, rice and leeks on the next day for lunch. You would only be testing the leeks at that time, but if you got any reaction, you would know it must be the leeks.

If you do get a reaction, you should not test a new food until you feel well again, otherwise you could mess up the whole test. You might have to wait anything up to three days. If you do get a certain reaction, it is wise to re-test that food, but not for at least another five days, or more.

If you break the diet once, you might have to start all over again. It means sticking to each day's foods rigidly and eating nothing else – no sauces, flavourings, etc.

Note: This food allergy test contains many foods with saturated fat. You may feel it is worthwhile including them in the test to see what kind of reaction you do get to them. Cut the fat off the lamb during the first five days. If you are taking dietary supplements watch out for additives to them like sugar or yeast. Gelatin-covered capsules can be taken throughout the test.

Isolating the Allergen

The important thing about testing foods one by one is that it isolates individual ingredients. You may, for example, feel ill after eating a piece of cake – but what is it in the cake that is making you feel bad? It could be the cane sugar, or the white flour, or the butter, or indeed the cherries on the top.

With bread, you could find that you are allergic to the yeast, rather than the wheat. Be particularly careful about sugar. Beet sugar and cane sugar are not the same thing, and you could react differently to each.

Do not think that foods must be safe because they are 'natural'. It is possible for tomatoes, potatoes, bananas, almonds, or peanuts, for example, to give you an allergic reaction, even though they are not refined or processed, or in any way adulterated.

Needless to say, the process of testing for food allergies is almost impossible socially. If you go out anywhere it is safest to take a picnic of 'safe' foods with you, and explain the reason to your host. It is too risky eating out as you do not know what the well-meaning cook might have added in the way of sauces.

You must also avoid all alcoholic drinks, you must not smoke, and take no drugs whatsoever. It is also a sensible idea to let your GP know what you are doing, but do not be surprised if he or she takes it less than seriously. Most doctors are not convinced by the food allergy theory.

Once you have avoided a troublemaker food for several days, you will react much more strongly to it when you do eat it again. This is a good way of double-testing the suspect foods. Even though these foods give you a bad time, do not be surprised if you also long for them – the two together are a sure sign. Once you have isolated the foods to which you are allergic, you should ideally give them up completely. If this is impossible, you could try being 'desensitized'.

Desensitization

The principle of desensitization is to find a dilution of the food to which the person is allergic which will 'switch off' the allergic reaction to that particular food.

Generally speaking, practitioners of environmental and nutritional medicine prefer MS patients to exercise self-control and avoid the offending foods completely. However, desensitization is a possibility in certain cases.

Rotation Diets

Giving up all the foods to which you are allergic is not quite enough. You also need to vary the remaining foods, and make sure you don't always eat the same thing day in, day out. This is called rotation dieting. Try not to eat one food within three days of having eaten it before. This lessens the chance of developing an allergy to new foods.

Some doctors who practise environmental medicine will allow a prohibited food to be carefully re-introduced after it has been avoided for six to nine months, on the proviso that it is only eaten as part of a rotation diet, and not with daily repetition. If you go back to old, addictive eating habits you could develop masked sensitivity.

OTHER WAYS OF TESTING FOR FOOD ALLERGIES

Around the UK there is now a group of doctors trained in orthodox medicine but who have been attracted by certain aspects of alternative medicine. These are the doctors trained in environmental and nutritional medicine. Because it is not taken seriously by the NHS, all these doctors practise privately. They take the concept of food allergies very seriously, and have some novel techniques to test for food and chemical sensitivities. Sometimes they use one technique, or a combination of testing techniques. New techniques involving one blood test are presently being developed.

The testing techniques they use seem a bit way-out, and it is hard to understand them. One is called the Vega test.

Vega Test

The Vega test works on the principles of Bio-Energetic Regulatory Medicine. It looks at the body from an electrical (bio-energetic) sense. It combines aspects of both acupuncture and homoeopathy.

The Vega test uses a machine about the size of a hi-fi amplifier. It has buttons, an indicator and a wire connected to a hand-held electrode and a measuring stylus.

The aim is to place into the machine glass phials containing homoeopathic doses of substances (e.g. possibly offending foods and chemicals) and find out if these substances are affecting the patient. The patient is given a hand-held cylinder to complete the electrical circuit. As each substance is put into the machine, the operator applies a tiny electrical current via an electrode to a point on the end of a finger or toe. This corresponds with known acupuncture points.

A bleep emits from the machine. If the bleep is low, it indicates that the substance is having a bad effect on the patient's condition.

Also, there is a lower reading than normal on the indicator dial.

If the sound of the bleep is normal, and the reading on the indicator dial is normal, then the person is not allergic to that particular substance.

This is a relatively fast and painless way of pinpointing the substances that are toxic to you.

The other new method which also seems crazy beyond belief is called applied kinesiology – but it really does seem to work.

Applied Kinesiology

Applied Kinesiology also works on the principles of Bio-Energetic Regulatory Medicine.

It tests the reaction of muscles as a way of detecting food allergies and nutrient imbalances.

The patient is asked to hold in his left hand a glass phial containing a homoeopathic dose of a particular substance. The patient will not know what this substance is. (Sometimes the phial is placed on the patient's stomach.) The practitioner will ask the patient to raise his right arm into the air, and to resist any pressure put on it by the practitioner.

If the patient is not allergic to the substance in the phial he will be able to resist the pressure on his right arm from the practitioner. The muscles in his arm will remain strong and of good tone, and he will have no trouble keeping his arm up in the air. The strength in his muscles suggests he needs the substance.

But if the substance given to the patient is toxic to him, he will be unable to resist the pressure of the practitioner on his right arm, and the arm will feel weak and the muscles lacking in tone, and he will give way under the pressure. The weakness in his muscles suggests he does not need this substance.

The practitioner of applied kinesiology gives the patient a succession of glass phials, each containing a substance. By putting pressure on the muscles of the raised arm, it is possible to identify those foods and substances to which the patient is allergic.

Many doctors do find applied kinesiology quite unbelievable – more like something out of a magic show than real medicine. But even so, many doctors who were once sceptical have now had to admit that, crazy though it sounds, it does work.

Applied kinesiology has been put to some scientific testing in the

USA. There was recently a report in the *Journal of Orthomolecular Psychiatry*[2] stating that muscle testing is an accurate, reliable and speedy method for determining food allergies.

As well as being a way of testing for food allergies, applied kinesiology can also be a treatment itself (see chapter 10).

Cytotoxic testing

Live white blood cells are exposed to a number of foods and chemicals. If the cells are damaged, this is a sign of sensitivity. The extent to which the cells are damaged gives an indication of the extent of the sensitivity. If there is no damage to the white blood cells, the substance being tested is harmless to that individual.

Intradermal Injection Techniques

This involves injecting tiny amounts of the allergen just beneath the skin surface. A weal – a small round bump – appears. If the weal gets bigger, it suggests an allergy to the substance. If the weal stays the same size, there is no allergy.

There are other diagnostic techniques to test for food allergies, but these are the main ones.

Nutritional Profile

Practitioners of environmental and nutritional medicine like to know the nutritional profile of each patient first by doing various tests. Hair analysis is widely used. Some doctors also use the sweat test, which is a very sophisticated test able to detect the nutritional status of a patient extremely accurately. These tests almost always show that an MS patient is low in zinc.

The nutritional supplements often prescribed by these practitioners are covered in detail in the previous chapter.

Certain amino acids are also prescribed.

Some doctors find that once the food allergies have been dealt with, and also the other problems, such as mercury toxicity or

2. Scopp, A. 'An experimental evaluation of kinesiology in allergy and deficiency disease diagnosis.' Vol. 7, 2, 137-138.

candidiasis, the nutrient balance in the body also sorts itself out to the extent that supplements are no longer necessary.

Conclusions

From work being done by some doctors both in the UK and the USA, it seems that food allergies should be taken very seriously by anyone with MS. The percentage of people with MS who improve once they avoid the foods to which they are allergic is very impressive.

SUCCESSES WITH EXCLUSION DIETS

The Roger MacDougall Diet

The best known and best publicized examples of people with MS whose lives changed as a result of identifying their food sensitivities are Roger MacDougall and Alan Greer.

Roger MacDougall lived until his 80s. Up until his death he was still fully mobile with good co-ordination and mobility. In 1953 he was firmly diagnosed as having MS and showed many of the classic symptoms. Within a few years of diagnosis his eyesight, legs, fingers and speech were badly affected. Before long, he was in a wheelchair. Without any medical training (he was a playwright and was professor in the University of California's Theatre department), Roger MacDougall decided to set about finding ways of treating his degenerative condition.

By a mixture of inspiration, guesswork, research, shots in the dark, and borrowing from other dietary regimes for MS, Roger MacDougall devised his own diet for MS. It began being just a gluten-free diet, but has evolved from that time to also virtually exclude sugar and dairy produce. It was also high in poly-unsaturated fats and low in saturated fats, and it had a long list of vitamin, mineral, trace element, and other supplements including polyunsaturates.

Roger MacDougall's diet used to be known as the 'Gluten-Free Diet' when it was first devised, but this is now a serious misnomer. Over the years, Roger MacDougall moved with the times, and his original diet evolved quite considerably.

It has four equally important elements:

1. No gluten.
2. Low sugar and no refined sugar.
3. Low milk products/high polyunsaturates.
4. Supplements of vitamins, minerals and trace elements, etc.

MacDougall first singled out gluten, which is the elastic-type stuff in dough. In coeliac disease, the sufferer is allergic to gluten. MacDougall thought this could also be happening in MS. The reasons why he linked MS with coeliac disease is because in coeliac disease the patient cannot assimilate fats. However, once wheat, barley, oats and rye are removed totally from the diet, fats can be taken into the body without any problem. MacDougall suggests that foods containing gluten 'damage the lining of the small intestine in such a way that the nutrients required to keep renewing the myelin sheath are prevented from reaching the bloodstream'.

In coeliac disease, the mucosal lining of the bowel is damaged so nutrients cannot be absorbed properly. MacDougall wondered if people with MS were experiencing something similar in their gut.

Sugar was excluded because of its role in causing hypoglycaemia, which can happen with MS. And as for dairy produce, its connection with the geographical distribution of MS was well known, and this was the same world map as for cardiovascular disease. The list of vitamins, minerals, trace elements and other supplements makes up for all the nutrients you would be deprived of if you gave up all cereals and dairy produce.

Gluten

Excluding gluten means excluding all foods containing wheat, barley, oats, and rye. This wipes out nearly all bread, cakes, biscuits, crispbreads, pasta, many breakfast cereals, and vast numbers of tinned and processed foods – look on the labels.

Recently, researchers from the National Institute of Mental Health in Washington found that gluten gives rise to substances called opioids in the gut. Some people cannot digest these, and researchers have found that they may block the conversion of dihomo-gammalinolenic acid to prostaglandins series 1.

An Australian doctor, Dr R Shatin from Melbourne, has

suggested that the demyelination of the nerve sheaths is secondary to an intolerance of gluten in the small intestine. He also put forward the hypothesis that the high rate of MS in Canada, Scotland, and Western Ireland may be due to the predominating use of Canadian wheat, which has the highest content of gluten of any in the world.

The cereals you can eat after you have excluded gluten are rice, maize (corn) and millet. You can safely use products such as rice flour, cornflour, breakfast cereals made with rice and corn (no added sugar), sago, tapioca. But of course these would only be OK if you were not allergic to any of them. (It is quite common to be allergic to corn.)

Sugar

Excluding sugar means eating nothing made from refined sugar or any product containing it, e.g. jams, marmalades, cakes, biscuits, tinned fruit, sweets, chocolate, ice cream, most drinks, processed foods, etc.

For sweetness, you could eat honey, raw Barbados sugar (not demerara), raw sugar chocolate, fructose, all fruit and dried fruits. (Make sure you are not *allergic* to sugar, though.)

Fat

Cut out butter, cream, full-cream milk, high fat cheeses. Do not eat fatty meats like bacon, pork, duck, goose, or processed meats like sausages.

Use only polyunsaturated margarine. (But watch out for whey, which is a milk product.) For cooking and salad dressing, use sunflower seed oil or safflower seed oil.

You can use small quantities of skimmed milk, low-fat cottage cheese, low-fat yogurt, eggs.

Offal meats like liver, kidneys, tongue, sweetbreads and brain can all be eaten. So can free-range animals such as venison, rabbit, poultry. *Lean* cuts of meat like beef, or pork are OK.

Drinks

Many drinks contain either gluten or sugar or both. Give up beer, whisky, gin, instant coffee, drinking chocolate, malted drinks, fizzy drinks, etc. Instead drink natural sugar-free fruit and vegetable juices, tea, decaffeinated coffee, mineral waters.

Other Foods

All other foods not on the exclusion list are OK to eat, e.g. all vegetables and legumes, pulses, seeds, nuts, all fish, all herbs, spices and condiments (use only natural essences and flavourings).

These are permitted on the Roger MacDougall diet because none of these things contain gluten, sugar or saturated fat. But if you believe in the principle of food allergy, it would be possible for you to be allergic to any of the above, e.g. tomatoes, bananas, or peanuts.

Supplements of Vitamins, Minerals, Trace Elements

This is necessary because cutting out so many grains and dairy produce also cuts out many other nutrients. So the vitamins, minerals and trace elements have to be replaced.

Roger MacDougall's list of supplements is remarkably similar to the list described in the previous chapters.

Vitamins

B vitamins: choline bitartrate, vitamin B1, vitamin B2, vitamin B6, folic acid, inositol, nicotinamide, pantothenic acid
Vitamin C
Vitamin E

Lipids

Lecithin, evening primrose oil, fish oil

Minerals and trace elements

Magnesium
Zinc

Copper
Iron
Selenium

Roger MacDougall has quite a considerable following, and receives heartening letters from people who have followed his dietary guidelines and improved.

His diet excludes a number of foods, any one (or more) of which could be causing allergy problems. Indeed, the reason why the Roger MacDougall diet may be working in so many people is because the excluded foods include some of the most common allergenic foods.

Rather than go on such a rigid diet, another approach would be to test yourself first for food allergies. It would be a pity to give up *all* grains if you were only found to be allergic to say, wheat.

Cutting down – or cutting out – sugar is good advice. But there are two distinct types of sugar – cane and beet. If you get yourself tested, you may find you are allergic to one but not the other.

It's a similar story with milk – cutting down on full-cream milk is good advice. However, milk is the most common allergenic food for people with MS. If you were tested for milk allergy, it would not help to continue taking any kind of milk at all, even skimmed milk or low-fat yogurts or cheeses.

There are several clinics around the UK which specialize in testing for food and environmental allergies. They are run by doctors who practise privately because what they do is not available on the National Health Service. To find your nearest doctor, your own GP should write to: British Society for Allergy, Environmental and Nutritional Medicine (BSAEM) (see Useful Addresses). They have a list of 150 doctors around the UK. Some have more experience treating MS than others.

Dr Bob Lawrence, a doctor who himself has MS, has devised a system of treating MS involving diet and nutritional supplements which he calls the ZENWA method, a Japanese term meaning balanced, harmonious diet. Details from:

Dietary Research Ltd.
Gwynfa House
10 Heol Gerrig
Treboeth
Swansea SA5 9BP
Tel: 01792 791081

The Rita Greer Diet

The other well-publicized case of an exclusion diet with a successful outcome is the Rita Greer Diet.

Rita Greer began experimenting with foods for her husband Alan at a time when he was severely disabled and doctors had written him off as a hopeless case.

Rita Greer told me recently: 'Alan has had MS for 36 years now. There is no doubt his diet and exercise programme and lifestyle keep the MS down to a minimum. Seeing he would be ''dead before he was 40'' forecast by 10 doctors, he's done well to reach 56.'

Rita's first breakthrough was when she accidentally discovered that Alan felt better on a diet which totally excluded meat – something she was forced to do through sheer poverty. From that, it was a short step to discover that he reacted badly to eggs and cheese, and all saturated fat.

Rita also decided to follow the principles of the gluten-free diet, and cut out everything made with wheat, barley, oats and rye.

By this time (early 1970s), sunflower seed oil was gaining popularity as a supplement for MS patients. So she began by giving her husband large daily doses of sunflower seed oil. But as soon as 'Naudicelle' became available, she replaced sunflower seed oil with these capsules of evening primrose oil.

With much trial and error, hard work, studying nutrition, and with the creativity that goes with being a gifted artist, she eventually came up with a diet that suited Alan. She kept him on this basically vegan diet for about four years, during which time he made gigantic improvements to the point where the wheelchair and walking aids were banished with the bedpans to the lumber room.

At the time of writing, when Alan is 56, he no longer has the relapsing/remitting type of MS, but the slow deterioration kind. He is still not in a wheelchair. His main MS symptoms now are a weak left hand and left leg, and sensitivity to light.

Rita Greer had an easy task finding out which foods made Alan worse – he was sick if he ate something he was allergic to. This is a very dramatic response and allergic reactions are usually more subtle than this.

The list of foods to which Rita found Alan was allergic *may not be the same list* for anyone else with MS.

His list of allergic foods was as follows:

Butter	Wheat	Cane sugar
cheese	barley	honey
milk	oats	jam
cream	rye	treacle
yogurt	and everything	sweets
lard	made with them	chocolate
eggs	such as bread,	
meat	pasta, biscuits,	
fatty fish like	cakes, breakfast	
herring and tuna	cereals, custard	
shellfish	powder)	
Drinking chocolate	Tinned fruit	Packaged,
malted drinks	tinned vegetables	tinned and
cocoa	bananas	processed
coffee	avocado pears	foods
strong tea	peanuts	semolina
squashes	brazil nuts	stock cubes
cordials	hazelnuts	spreads and
spirits	chestnuts	pastes.
alcoholic drinks		

Alan also gave up smoking.

He took supplements of evening primrose oil, multi-vitamin and mineral tablets, and vitamin B12 (essential for non-meat-eaters).

Even though he excluded many foods, this still left him with a wide choice, especially of fruits and vegetables, and white fish.

However, there is no guarantee that the fruits and vegetables which were perfectly OK for Alan Greer would not cause reactions in someone else with MS.

Full details of the Greer diet can be found in *Diets to Help Multiple Sclerosis* by Rita Greer, published by Thorsons.

More recently, the film director Bryan Forbes has gone on record as having greatly improved his MS symptoms by going on a diet which excludes wheat, barley, oats and rye, and by taking vitamin supplements. His wife, actress Nanette Newman, dreamed up delicious recipes which excluded all these grains. (See *A Divided Life* by Bryan Forbes, published by Heinemann.)

The conclusion from all of these is to get yourself tested for your own personal food allergies before copying what someone else did. What worked for them might not work for you, and it would be foolish to go on these difficult diets if they are not tailor-made for your needs.

The Multiple Sclerosis Healing Trust has weekly clinics where people with MS can see a doctor specializing in nutritional and environmental medicine. They also offer massage, shiatsu, reflexology, magnetotherapy and counselling.

Multiple Sclerosis Healing Trust
PO Box 2469
Shirley
Solihull
West Midlands B90 2QZ
Tel: 0121-422 6162 or 0121-733 8982

Many MS Therapy Centres include nutrition advice (see Useful Addresses).

10

Holistic Medicine

Many therapies which come under the broad heading of holistic or alternative medicine can be very helpful in MS. This includes not only the well-established therapies such as acupuncture, osteopathy, and homoeopathy, but also the newer ones such as aromatherapy, applied kinesiology, electro-magnetic therapy, and reflexology.

Many of the holistic therapies share some of the concepts of the ancient Eastern systems of medicine in which balance is synonymous with good health. Good health is harmony: a balance between opposing forces, between yin and yang, or between acid and alkaline.

Harmony also involves much more than just a biochemical balance. As in the traditional Eastern forms of medicine, it also means right life, wisdom and love, right fellowship, meditation, healthy eating and exercise.

No matter what therapy you are talking about, any kind of alternative therapy is likely to be holistic in its approach. Unlike the orthodox doctor, the alternative therapist will attempt to treat you as a whole person – mind, body and spirit – and not just the diseased part. This holistic approach also extends to the treatment itself, which can encompass every aspect of a person's life, and not just their physical symptoms.

In fact, the whole approach of all the alternative therapies is radically different from that of orthodox medicine. By and large, they are not very interested in giving diseases labels such as multiple sclerosis or arthritis. Broadly, they tend to view disease as a loss of balance in the body, brought about by an imbalanced lifestyle and thought patterns.

They also tend to believe that, with help, the body can be brought back into balance and that good health can be regained – in other words, healing can take place. They generally do not go along with the concept of 'incurable' diseases. Although none would claim to 'cure' MS, many do say that the condition can be stabilized and that the downward spiral can be stopped or even reversed.

Orthodox medicine diagnoses symptoms and tries to find ways of suppressing those symptoms, usually through drugs. By contrast, holistic therapists aim not to suppress symptoms, but to get to the root cause or causes of the symptoms, and to treat those root causes instead.

The general starting point with alternative medicine is the conviction that the body has innate powers to heal itself, given the right conditions. The task of any alternative therapist is to help bring about the right conditions so the body can get on with the business of healing itself.

The mistake some patients make is to view a particular alternative therapy as just a technique. This is a very conventional, as well as passive view of medicine.

If you want any kind of holistic therapy to be helpful, you have to be an active participant in the healing process, and not just a passive recipient, who has something done to you.

Before you go and see any holistic practitioner (which includes some trained 'orthodox' doctors) you should be psychologically prepared to fundamentally change many aspects of your life. The therapy itself is likely to be only one part of a holistic treatment program which may involve quite dramatic changes to diet, lifestyle, exercise and thought patterns.

The whole attitude of holistic medicine transforms your way of thinking, and makes you think seriously about how *you* came to have MS. You may well, with the help of the therapist, discover aspects of your old lifestyle which have to be changed now if you want to get better and not worse.

So getting involved in alternative medicine may well mean making radical changes to your life, your lifestyle, how you eat, what you eat, what you drink, and the way you think. But the approach of alternative medicine is very positive and hopeful, as you no longer classify yourself in the orthodox mode of being someone with an incurable illness. Instead, you see yourself as someone who is making profound changes to help regain health.

Is Alternative Therapy Effective?

There are claims from many holistic therapists that what they do can help MS. They never use the word 'cure', as this is not the way they think. It is difficult to be precise about to what extent they can be effective. This differs from case to case. It is always hard to turn the clock back, and reverse existing damage. But some already-disabled people may well feel increased well-being as a result of seeing a holistic practitioner; and someone with only mild MS symptoms may find that these symptoms do go away with treatment. Everyone, no matter what their degree of the disease, should experience a greater sense of well-being as a result of treatment in the chosen therapy, together with some lifestyle changes.

What Alternative Therapy?

In this book I do not intend to go into detail about what all the various alternative or holistic therapies consist of; how they work and what they do. There are several good books which do that. An excellent one is *The Natural Family Doctor* edited by Dr Andrew Stanway, published by Century.

Which therapy, or therapies, you choose may depend on what appeals to you most, or which one has been recommended to you, or what is available in your area.

Many of them are trying to achieve the same ends by different means.

I have had a good personal experience of several of them, and they may have played a part in stabilizing my condition. These are specifically: acupuncture, osteopathy, hydrotherapy, herbalism, applied kinesiology, massage, reflexology, and electro-magnetic therapy.

Nearly all of the alternative therapies have experience of treating patients with multiple sclerosis.

These are (in no particular order):

Homoeopathy
Herbalism
Aromatherapy
Naturopathy
Hydrotherapy
Osteopathy
Cranial Osteopathy
Chiropractic
Massage
Applied Kinesiology
Reflexology
Acupuncture
Shiatsu
Alexander Technique
Healing
Meditation (see also chapter 15)
Electro-magnetic therapy.

Quite often, if you see one therapist, he or she may refer you to another therapy or therapies if he or she feels you could benefit from another approach as well.

I believe it is worth getting involved in the whole field of holistic medicine, at the very least because it transforms your attitudes and your lifestyle to healthier ones. And at the very best, it can improve your health.

11

Mercury in Dental Fillings

Is MS a Reaction to Environmental Toxins?

Some doctors working in the field of environmental medicine believe that degenerative diseases such as multiple sclerosis are a sort of slow poisoning of the system.

Everyday things in our environment which are harmless to most people prove to be toxic to some susceptible people. The people who are susceptible to environmental toxins seem to have a poorer ability to adapt than others.

Case histories of patients who have been treated in this field show that if they are exposed to certain environmental toxins their symptoms get worse, but when these toxins are taken away, the symptoms get better.

Food has already been discussed in some detail. The other things which can be toxic to people with MS are a whole range of chemicals found in our everyday lives, and also certain metals. Chemicals are discussed in the second half of this chapter.

Of all the metals which can be toxic to someone with MS, mercury is probably the worst. Dr Patrick Kingsley is convinced that mercury is the underlying cause of MS.

Mercury is a toxic metal. Yet it has been used in amalgam dental fillings for more than a century.

Recently, there has been growing concern that some of this mercury could be seeping into the body, causing serious health problems, sometimes including neurological symptoms.

The people who have dared raise their voices against mercury in dental fillings are a few dentists, nutritionists, and a handful of doctors both here and in the USA. They are up against the majority of the dental and medical establishment who insist that the mercury in fillings is safe and who take the view that linking MS symptoms to the mercury in your fillings is unproven and irresponsible.

This heated controversy is still being aired in the dental and medical literature.

THE CASE AGAINST MERCURY

Mercury is one of the most toxic poisons known to humanity. When it was first used as a component in fillings, dentists thought it was safe because it was used together with other metals.

What Fillings Are Made of

Pure mercury (also known as quicksilver) is mixed with particles of silver, copper, and tin to form a putty-like mix. This mix – or amalgam – is placed in the tooth. The mercury hardens and holds these particles together.

Mercury Can Get Into the Body

Because mercury was mixed with these other metals, it was thought to be stable. But mercury in amalgam fillings is not stable. Mercury, in a variety of forms, can get into the body. It can leak into the tooth or gum; you can swallow it with saliva; you can breathe it in.

Over the years, mercury seeps from fillings in minute amounts. How much mercury seeps out depends on how much dental plaque there is, the pH (acid/alkaline balance) inside the mouth, how old the fillings are, how many fillings you have, how hard you chew, what food you eat, your individual body chemistry, and so on.

As well as the chronic low-level exposure, every day, for years on end, there is also acute exposure to mercury vapour when you are having a filling put in or taken out.

Elemental mercury gives off a vapour when it is agitated, compressed, heated, or exposed to air at normal temperature. It is easy to breathe this vapour in. It goes through the thin bony plates at the top of the mouth, into the sinuses, into the orbit of the eye, and the chambers of the inner ear where the body's balancing mechanism is situated. It also gets into the brain, which is so near the top of the mouth. And it also goes into the temporomandibular joint which controls the functions of the jaw. Mercury vapour also gets into the lungs.

Various biological processes inside the body transform mercury vapour into methylmercury, which is 100 times more toxic than mercury vapour.

Mercury vapour can mix with food. When it gets into the stomach, mercury can react with hydrochloric acid, resulting in the formation of mercuric chloride. This can create a shortage of hydrochloric acid, which means that food cannot be digested properly.

Fillings Provide a Continuous Source of Mercury

Even though your body will be excreting mercury (which is measurable), some mercury will remain in your system. How much mercury is there, where exactly it is, and what it is doing to you are far less easy to measure.

If you have several fillings in your mouth, you have a continuous source of mercury. This means that in the course of a lifespan, mercury will be accumulated in almost every organ.

Research has shown that amalgam fillings do not remain the same as the day they were put in, and that there is a substantial loss of mercury. In the USA, researchers found an astonishingly high loss of mercury compared with the original filling. What this means is that you could have ingested anything between 30 to 560mg of mercury particles or vapour over the years, depending on the number of fillings you have. On a day-to-day basis, this is a very small amount of mercury, but even tiny amounts of mercury can be damaging.

Fillings will corrode in time. This corrosion is partly because fillings are subjected to all the chemicals put into the mouth, both from food and drink and those produced by your own body. But the corrosion is also partly due to electrical activity.

Mercury from corroded amalgam fillings can get into the body. You can inhale the vapour, or swallow or convert the particles that result from corrosion.

Your Mouth Is Like an Electrical Generator

If you have more than one kind of metal in your mouth, then you have electricity in your mouth. This is because all metals are reservoirs of energy called electrons. If electrons can flow through some kind of conductor, then you have an electrical current. Saliva is an electrolyte (an aqueous solution with metal ions capable of transporting an electrical current).

This electrical activity can cause corrosion of fillings. It can also affect the function of cranial nerves, which in itself can affect any system in the body.

Where Does Mercury Inside Your Body Go?

Mercury can go everywhere – it is able to travel all over the body, upsetting intricate processes.

Primarily, mercury affects the central nervous system. It can also cause particular havoc on the immune system. Mercury can inactivate the lymphocytes, and alter the ratio between 'T' suppressor and 'T' helper cells.

Mercury can also accumulate in the kidneys, heart muscle, lungs, liver, brain and red blood cells. Other areas where mercury can be stored are the thyroid gland, pituitary gland, adrenal glands, spleen, testes, bone marrow, and intestinal wall. Mercury can get through the blood–brain barrier and enter the nerve cells from the blood, destroying nerve tissue as it does so.

What Damage Does Mercury Do?

Most people are not affected by the mercury in their fillings – not overtly, anyway. But some people are.

As mercury is capable of damaging many tissues and organs, thereby disturbing their normal functions, it is not surprising that the list of symptoms which can be caused by mercury poisoning is very long.

A general list includes:

Bleeding gums, increased salivation, sour-metallic taste, facial paralysis, irregular heartbeat, depression, strong pains in the left part of chest, retinal bleeding, dim vision, uncontrollable eye movement, irritability, vertigo, headaches, joint pains, pains in the lower back, stress intolerance, decreased sexual activity, Bell's Palsy.

Specifically neurological symptoms include:

Mild tremor, ataxia (lack of muscle co-ordination and irregular movement), sensory loss, visual problems, fatigue, numbness and tingling of hands, feet, lips, muscle weakness progressing to paralysis, speech disorders, general central nervous system dysfunctions.

Mercury has a devastating effect on the body's immune system, particularly on the 'T' cells which have a vital part to play in cell-mediated immunity. This means that mercury can alter the body's defence mechanisms against infection and disease, and also make people more prone to allergy. In addition, mercury may cause vascular damage to the brain and spinal cord. MS is now considered by many to be primarily a vascular disorder.

MERCURY IN FILLINGS AND MULTIPLE SCLEROSIS

Is multiple sclerosis mercury poisoning? Do some of the neurological symptoms from mercury poisoning mimic multiple sclerosis? Are people with MS especially sensitive to mercury? Or does mercury simply enhance MS symptoms?

Both in the UK and USA, there have been several documented cases of people who were told they had MS, had their fillings removed, and whose 'MS' symptoms went away. For example, in his book about mercury/amalgam dental fillings, *The Toxic Time Bomb*, (Thorsons), author Sam Ziff describes some such cases, and the British media have also highlighted a few cases. Did these people really have MS? Or did their symptoms just seem like MS? Or was their MS made worse by the mercury poisoning? The general view amongst the doctors and dentists who believe there is a connection between mercury and MS say that mercury can exacerbate MS symptoms, or mimic MS, but it does *not* actually *cause* MS. They believe there is already a predisposition to MS, which was there before any fillings were put in.

In some cases, it seems that the neurological symptoms mimic multiple sclerosis, and that therefore the diagnosis of MS is a mistaken one.

London dentist Vicky Lee says,

'Many patients with MS have been diagnosed only on clinical symptoms, and these symptoms may be identical with heavy metal poisoning – in particular mercury poisoning with symptoms such as tremor, ataxia, irritability, fatigue, cold sweats, frequent urination and eye symptoms.'

The Hypothesis that Mercury Poisoning Leads to MS

However, there are some people who believe that mercury in fillings *is* a cause of MS. In 1983 an article entitled 'Epidemiology, Etiology, and Prevention of Multiple Sclerosis' written by Theodore H. Ingalls, MD, of the Epidemiology Study Center in Framingham, Massachusetts, was published in the American *Journal of Forensic Medicine and Pathology* (vol. 4, number 1, March 1983). It began:

Slow, retrograde seepage of ionic mercury from root canal or . . . amalgam fillings inserted many years previously, recurrent caries and corrosion around filling edges, and the oxidizing effect of the purulent response may lead to multiple sclerosis in middle age.

Dr Ingalls, himself an MS sufferer, goes on to say that the world map of MS could be explained by the greater incidence of dental caries in the parts of the world where MS is high, and the lower incidence of dental caries in those parts of the world where MS is low. Obviously, the more dental caries there are, the more fillings there are. He suggests that perhaps dental caries are a precursor of MS. As well as mercury, Dr Ingalls thinks that lead may also be involved in MS:

Clinical and epidemiologic data also suggest that a second heavy metal, lead, may operate almost interchangeably with mercury. Possibly, cases of unilateral (one side only) MS derive from mercury – amalgam fillings in teeth, whereas the generalized disease may result from ingestion or inhalation of volatile mercury or exhaust fumes of lead additives to gasoline (petrol).

He also argues that heavy metal poisoning may be coming from other sources apart from tooth fillings.

Heavy Metal Poisoning from Farming and Industrial Techniques

Certain fungicides and weedkillers contain mercury. Perhaps this is a factor which might help explain why MS is higher in farming rather than fishing areas. Mercury is also found in some industrial germicides.

SHOULD YOU HAVE YOUR FILLINGS REMOVED?

This question is not as simple as it seems. Not everyone with MS is necessarily reacting to the mercury in their fillings. No one has been taking reliable statistics, but it seems that more than half of those people with MS who have been tested for mercury sensitivity show positive results. If you are positive to mercury, then it would be worth having your fillings out. It would not be worth having your fillings taken out if you show no sensitivity to mercury.

There are certain tests which can indicate whether or not you are hypersensitive to mercury. One, using an electrical meter, measures the electrical activity in the mouth. The other methods are the Vega test, and applied kinesiology (see chapter on food allergies). To have these tests, you would have to find a private dentist or a clinical ecologist, as they are not available on the NHS.

To find one, write to the Dental Society for Clinical Nutrition. The president is Jack Levenson. He can be contacted at:

No. 1 Welbeck House
62 Welbeck Street
London W1M 7HB
Tel: 0171-486 3127

Dangers in the Removal of Fillings

The removal of fillings is not a simple matter, and there are dangers in the procedure.

The danger with removing fillings is that mercury vapour is

released into the air. There seems to be little disagreement that the highest levels of mercury vapour are reached during the insertion and removal of amalgam, with a potential danger to both the patient and the dental practitioner. Some dentists are willing to place a full-mouth rubber dam in the mouth which prevents mercury vapour from escaping. As an extra precaution, they might take out only a few fillings at a time instead of several or even all of them. This would make the removal of a large number of fillings a lengthy procedure as well as an expensive one.

However, there is no doubt that some people with MS have had very dramatic improvements after their fillings had gone. But as well as the more publicized cases of people with MS whose symptoms have disappeared after the removal of their fillings, there are also those cases where the MS has worsened after a full-scale removal of fillings.

So the first thing to do is find a sympathetic dentist, get yourself tested, and then follow his or her advice. Even those dentists who believe there is an overwhelming connection between mercury in your fillings and MS may think it is better to leave them well alone if you show no sensitivity to mercury, and are in a stable condition. But it seems worth taking the risks involved if you do show a sensitivity to mercury, as improvements can be astounding. It is fair to say that the removal of fillings *may* help in MS, rather than *will* help.

MERCURY AND MICRONUTRIENTS

Many people with MS are low in zinc, manganese, chromium, molybdenum, selenium, and other trace elements. Of these, the most important is zinc (see chapter 8).

If you were to weigh the amount of mercury being placed in a large filling, there might be as much as 1 gram of mercury alone. There is potentially enough mercury in the mouth to interfere with the micronutrients of the body.

The amount of mercury released during the placement and removal of an amalgam filling is certainly enough to unbalance the very tiny amounts of micronutrients even in a healthy person, at least for a short time.

When the body is short of essential micronutrients it has a greater chance of being laid open to mercury poisoning. If there is a shortage of zinc and selenium, mercury cannot bind to zinc/selenium protein complexes. So mercury can rampage freely around the body, locked in because the mechanism for its removal is not there.

The body may be attempting to rid itself of mercury through the bile and sweat, but in fact may be re-absorbing it in the colon and through the skin, particularly if someone is not very physically active, cannot wash himself daily, and is constipated.

CAN YOU DETOXIFY YOURSELF OF MERCURY WITHOUT HAVING ALL YOUR FILLINGS REMOVED?

Nutritional methods on their own will not be sufficient to detoxify the body of mercury, although they will help.

If you have all the tests and you do show a sensitivity to mercury, then it is probably best to have your fillings taken out. But even after you have done this, there will still be mercury left in your body. The removal of fillings will get rid of about 50 per cent of the mercury. But that still leaves the other 50 per cent to be got rid of.

So you should follow up the removal of fillings with nutritional methods. Even if you don't show any sensitivity to mercury, and don't have your fillings removed, it would be a good idea to follow the same nutritional programme, which is designed to escort toxins out of the body.

It is possible that if you are having optimum nutrition, you can reverse a sensitivity to mercury as shown in the tests mentioned above.

Oral Chelation Therapy

The nutritional method which can help detoxify the body is called 'oral chelation therapy'. Chelation simply means latching on to something else. As well as helping to detoxify the body, oral chelation therapy is also a way of replacing essential nutrients which may be inactivated by low level chronic exposure to mercury.

Dr Patrick Kingsley, a doctor practising in Leicestershire, who has had great success with pinpointing and removing toxins from people with MS, likes to use tablets called 'Health Insurance Plus', made by Lamberts. They can be prescribed on the NHS if your doctor is willing, as they have not been put on the blacklist (i.e. drugs or preparations not prescribable on the NHS). Dr Kingsley recommends 2 tablets, 3 times a day, starting 7 days prior to the first dental amalgam removal and continuing for 6 weeks after the last amalgam has gone.

Apart from a wide range of essential vitamins and minerals, 'Health Insurance Plus' tablets contain 2 amino acids (cysteine and methionine) that have something called S-H bonds, known technically as sulphydril groups. These are particularly effective at latching onto toxic minerals such as lead or mercury. Once this latching-on process has happened, vitamin C (1 gram 3 times daily) will help to excrete these toxic metals from the body.

Sulphydril groups are also present in onions and garlic. These are also valuable in detoxifying the body. However, they should be avoided if you are on homoeopathic remedies, as they act as an antidote.

Information about the following nutrients which help to detoxify the body comes from *The Toxic Time Bomb,* written by Sam Ziff and published by Thorsons (now out of print).

Cysteine

The amino acid cysteine has a specific affinity for mercury and will bind with it, allowing excretion of it from the body. Vitamin C must be taken with cysteine at a ratio of 3:1. (Cysteine is in 'Health Insurance Plus' – see above).

Glutathione

Glutathione is composed of the amino acids cysteine, glutamic acid and glycine and serves as a storage and transport vehicle for cysteine. Glutathione is a water-soluble anti-oxidant and free radical scavenger and acts as a detoxicant against heavy metal toxins. It works with vitamins C and E, adding to their roles as anti-oxidants. The suggested dose is 50mg twice daily.

Vitamin C and Vitamin E

They are important agents against mercury because mercury is known to cause free radicals in the body, and these vitamins scavenge and mop up free radicals.

Research papers show that vitamin E can reduce the toxic effects of mercury. In laboratory tests, vitamin E was able to reduce the chromosomal breakage caused by mercury. The suggested dose of vitamin C is 1000-3000mg, and 100-400 i.u. of vitamin E.

Selenium and Molybdenum

Some studies have shown that selenium and molybdenum can reduce the toxic effects of mercury. Do not exceed 200 µg a day of selenium as it can be toxic.

Zinc

Mercury can displace zinc in the body. Yet zinc is a vital trace element to latch on to mercury and escort it out of the body. Suggested dose is 20-50mg a day.

Magnesium

Mercury can inhibit various enzyme systems in the body by inhibiting the activity of magnesium. Suggested dose 100-200mg per day. Be careful of creating an imbalance between magnesium and calcium. If necessary, take calcium supplements, or Dolomite, a mixture of calcium and magnesium carbonates.

Vitamin B6

Vitamin B6 is involved in how the body handles the detoxification of mercury. Suggested dose 50-200mg daily.

Rutin

Rutin is one of the bioflavonoid family. It seems to have a specificity for binding to and helping to remove mercury from the body.

Calcium Pantothenate or Pantothenic Acid

The physiologically active form of pantothenic acid is coenzyme A. Mercury can inhibit or suppress coenzyme A, which is also a co-factor involved in adrenal function. Pantothenic acid should be taken if fillings are removed, as this is an additional stress to the body. Dose 100-400mg daily.

Vitamin B1 (Thiamine)

Thiamine is important in the decarboxylation process of cellular respiration. There is a critical step at the entrance into the aerobic oxidation cycle. This step involves coenzyme A. Coenzyme A carries fatty acids to the membranes of the mitochondria and hands them over to the amino-acid carnitine, which crosses the inner membrane of the mitochondria. Carnitine then hands over the fatty acids to another molecule of coenzyme A. The mitochondria are the power centres of each cell. It is in the mitochondria that glucose and fatty acids are oxidized in order to generate the energy that powers us. Coenzyme A contains a sulphydril group (SH). These SH groups are susceptible to being inactivated by mercury and so unable to produce acetyl-coenzyme A.

Adding thiamine helps to repair the impaired area of the metabolic cycle. The limited amounts of coenzyme A still available are used more efficiently.

The dose of thiamine is 50mg morning and evening. It should be taken in a B complex tablet.

Acidophilus

Acidophilus is a friendly bacteria found in live yogurt which goes to make up intestinal flora. The intestinal flora may play a significant part in determining the excretion rate of mercury.

Candida (see chapter 9)

There is a relationship between candida and mercury. There seems to be a connection between the presence of amalgam and the body's ability to cope with yeast candida albicans. Candida is considered normal flora, but when the body's immune mechanisms are impaired, candida can increase until it produces disease-like symptoms. If you are sensitive to mercury, candida organisms are resistant to treatment. But once you get rid of mercury, the candida is more amenable to treatment.

Other Aspects of Multiple Sclerosis and Dentistry

Some holistic doctors have found that people with MS have a problem with their temporomandibular joint, which is a hinge joint in the jaw which articulates the mandible and the temporal bones. As a result, their teeth and bite are out of alignment. A cranial osteopath should be able to correct this.

Some people with MS have reported that once their temporomandibular joint was corrected there was an improvement in other MS symptoms. This correction can be done by either a skilled cranial osteopath, or a chiropractor trained in what they call 'sacro-occipital technique'.

Sacro-occipital technique is the technique of adjusting irregular bite. It describes itself as 'a system of removing the cause of nerve malfunction using minimum force to restore and maintain health'.

The thinking behind this technique is that when there are distortions in the skull, this has an effect on normal cerebro-spinal fluid flow and the nervous system.

12

Chemicals and Other Environmental Toxins

The list of chemicals and other environmental toxins which could affect someone with MS is very long indeed. It includes many of the things you probably take for granted in your everyday life, such as aerosol sprays, tap water, and even chipboard. More obvious toxins include lead from car exhaust fumes and – worse – diesel fumes. And, of course, cigarette smoke.

Many of these things, such as cosmetics made from coal tar or food with artificial colouring, you may have been used to for several years. So why do they only seem to be having a bad effect on you now? This could be because of Toxic Overload.

Toxic Overload

It seems that some people are better able to adapt to new stresses than others. The theory of General Adaptation Syndrome comes originally from Dr Theron Randolph, the founding father of Clinical Ecology in the USA.

Roughly, the theory goes like this. This syndrome begins with repeated occasional exposure to any irritant substance. At a certain level of exposure, the person has a rejection response, or 'alarm' response. The 'alarm' response will happen any time the person is exposed to the substance, as long as this exposure happens only now and again.

However, if the exposure happens more than occasionally, i.e. frequently or all the time, the response is different. The person appears to be adapted to the substance. This is the 'resistance' phase.

But this apparent adaptation is not a genuine adaptation at all. What in fact is going on is that the body is making a huge internal effort to cope with the stresses of the substance.

The body makes much larger quantities than usual of hormones such as cortisone and adrenalin. These hormones in the blood can give you a boost of energy and a feeling of well-being. But it is not long-lived, because after a short time these hormones are spent.

When this happens, the person may seek out the substance, like an addict. If this addiction is not satisfied, the adaptation breaks down. When this happens, the reaction to the substance becomes the 'alarm' response again, but in a more dramatic form.

The phase when the body's adaptive ability breaks down is called the 'exhaustion' phase. The affected person may feel ill or irritable all the time. The way out of this is to withdraw the offending substance from the person. At first, this may have the effect of making him more ill. But there is no other way to get the whole system back on an even keel.

A wide range of symptoms can be explained by this General Adaptation Syndrome. It also extends into behaviour, thinking, and personality. All these things can be caused by foods, chemicals, or metals.

It could be argued that anyone with MS has already reached the 'exhaustion' phase. If you can identify which things are causing *your* toxic overload, and if you can then remove these things from your life, there is the chance of getting better instead of getting worse.

Your own GP may well think this is all a bit far-fetched. You may need the help of a doctor trained in 'environmental medicine'. Ask your GP to write to the following address for a list of such doctors:

British Society for Allergy and Environmental Medicine (BSAEM)
PO Box 28
Totton
Southampton
SO40 2ZA

The clinics listed in the Useful Addresses chapter can test you for chemical and environmental toxins.

A very helpful book which goes into this subject in great detail is *Chemical Children* by Dr Peter Mansfield and Dr Jean Monro, published by Century paperbacks.

Chemicals in Foods

Be aware of chemicals in foods. Read labels like a hawk when you go shopping. With a new awareness, you can totally avoid chemicals in foods.

Unnatural, degraded, processed food may be a cause of degenerative diseases, of which MS is one. It is only in this century that a whole generation has grown up with eating food which has been adulterated.

Chemical fertilizers, pesticides and insecticides assault fruit, vegetables, and crops while they are growing. Steroids and antibiotics are given to intensively-reared livestock.

In the manufacturing process, a whole range of additives may be added to foods, including artificial colourings, flavourings, and preservatives.

In the last few years the public has been alerted to the 'E' additives in manufactured foods, and there has been a link made between certain 'E' numbers in foods, and hyperactivity in children.

However, the additives in foods may also be affecting people who have MS. Chemicals which are taken in food and drink (or breathed in) can soon produce allergic-type responses.

Even food that you think looks perfectly 'natural' may have been polluted before it reaches you, the consumer. In fact, the more perfect the specimen of fruit or vegetable, the more suspicious of it you should be, because only fruit and vegetables which have been successfully protected (by chemicals) will be in 'perfect' condition by the time they reach the supermarket or greengrocer.

How to Avoid Chemicals In Foods

Do not buy anything which is processed. All junk food is out. Whatever you buy that does come out of a tin or a packet, at least read the label. If there are any additives, preservatives, colourings, flavourings – don't buy it.

As a rule, always try and buy pure, fresh things instead of

processed foods. The fresher the food is, the more 'alive' it is. Frozen food will have lost some of its goodness, and may have colouring in it, such as the bright green used on frozen peas.

If you can, switch to organic food. It is getting easier all the time to find places which sell organic food – not just organically grown fruit and vegetables, but also meat, poultry, bread, dried produce, etc. which are free of all chemicals.

To find out your nearest organic produce retailer write to:

The Soil Association Ltd.,
86 Colston Street,
Bristol BS1 5BB,
Tel: 0272 290661

or:

The Henry Doubleday Research Association,
Ryton-on-Dunsmore,
Coventry,
CV8 3LG.

Chemicals in Everyday Life

The most dangerous place to find chemicals which could affect your health is your own home. The chances are that every single room in your home will have things in it to which you could be reacting badly.

Here are just some of the baddies to look for:

Tap water. This contains chlorine, nitrates, possibly fluoride and polyphosphates.
Aerosol sprays, such as furniture polish, air freshener, fly spray, perfume, deodorant, etc. All aerosols use a liquid propellant. When you press the button, a spray of fine droplets of this propellant squirts out under the pressure of the gas in the can. This propellant liquid evaporates, leaving fine particles of the chemical in the air. The technical name for this kind of gas is halocarbon.
Fumes from gas boiler, stove, or fires if ventilation is bad.
Chipboard and foam in furniture. This gives off a type of gas called formaldehyde. Formaldehyde is also found in other common items in the home, such as the combustion products of natural gas,

tobacco smoke, glossy magazines and books, and newspapers.

There is a hypothesis that people with MS are grossly contaminated with formaldehyde. It comes from Mr RC Baskerville, who has written lengthy papers on the topic, but was denied a grant from any of the MS associations to do further research.

He can be contacted at:

Baskerville Technical Services,
1 Russell Close,
Stevenage, SG2 8PB

Other noxious chemicals in the home include:

- Plastics. Even though you can't see it, they give off a gas.
- Chemicals in cleaning agents, insect killers, weed killers, DDT, etc.
- Synthetic carpets and fabrics (which are treated with insecticide in the manufacturing process).
- All solvents – glues, typewriter correcting fluid, nail varnish, nail varnish remover, dry cleaning fluid, etc. Gloss paint.
- Cosmetics and toiletries made from coal tar products.
- Cosmetics and toiletries made with chemical colourants. Watch out for brightly coloured bath salts, coloured toilet paper, etc.
- Toothpaste containing fluoride and colouring. The adverse effects of fluoride include interference with a wide range of metabolic enzymes.

These chemicals can be inhaled through the airways, or be absorbed through the skin, or ingested. For example, watch out for washing up liquid on plates which have not been rinsed properly – the detergent can affect the stomach lining.

Unless you are obviously sensitive to these chemicals, for example you sneeze terribly if someone uses aerosol hair spray, you may not be aware that the gases given off by some of these products may be affecting you.

As well as halocarbon vapour from all sorts of aerosols, the same sort of gas comes from solvents used in cosmetics, glues, stain-removers, cleaning fluids, etc.

Other gases which are given off from common household things are acetone and ether, as well as formaldehyde which I have already mentioned.

All these gases dissolve into the air completely, leaving no haze. But just because you can't see them, it doesn't mean they are not having a toxic effect on you.

Chemical Pollutants Outside the Home

The worst chemical pollutants outside the home for someone with MS are diesel fumes, and lead from petrol exhaust fumes. So living in cities, or near traffic-clogged arterial routes, may be worse for you than living in a place with relatively clean air, such as the seaside.

These pollutants can also affect food on sale in greengrocers' shops which are situated on main roads near traffic lights. If the fruit and vegetables are displayed outside on the pavement in such a position, they are bound to be contaminated with the toxins given off by the traffic. The best thing is to avoid buying produce from such a shop.

Alternatives to Chemicals

It is possible to find alternatives to all of the noxious chemicals mentioned.

Cleaning Agents

Several brands are biodegradable. The range includes fabric softener, soap, and washing up liquid. Or use ordinary soda crystals. Buy tins of polish instead of aerosols.

Toothpaste

Use bicarbonate of soda instead, or a homoeopathic brand such as Toms or Neilsons.

Cosmetics and Toiletries

Use soap without colouring or scent, such as Simple soap and other similar products. Roc or Almay are also good. Use Aloe Vera shampoo and other cosmetics. Make sure there are no detergents and no additives.

Water

Buy a water filter which can be connected to your water mains and becomes like a 'third tap' in your kitchen. This filters out all the harmful substances in the mains drinking water supply. Alternatively, buy a jug filter, or use pure bottled spring water, such as Highland Spring or Malvern.

Furniture and Furnishings

Avoid chipboard. Avoid foam. Avoid synthetic fabrics. Go instead for solid wood, and natural fibres in cushions and mattresses, and also in fabrics for furnishings.

Bedding

As you spend about 8 hours out of every 24 in bed, it is important for the bed to be uncontaminated by chemical pollutants. Ideally, the frame should be metal, or hardwood. Even a wood like pine gives off fumes, called terpenes. Be careful about the headboard, and avoid anything with foam or chipboard. Try and get a mattress made with natural fibres. If you have a foam mattress, cover it with old-fashioned cotton ticking. Go for pure cotton sheets and pillow cases, and duvet covers if you have them. Avoid polyester, which is a synthetic and part of the plastics family.

Gas Appliances

Ideally, site the boiler in an outhouse, or else housed in a casing which will stop the fumes getting into the kitchen. If necessary, improve the ventilation.

Clothes

Avoid synthetic fabrics, and wool, which is often treated chemically. The best fabric is pure cotton. Avoid sending your clothes to the dry cleaners, as dry cleaning fluid gives off fumes. If you have to dry clean certain garments, air them thoroughly outdoors before wearing them. You could probably safely ignore some labels inside garments, and wash them though the label may say 'dry clean only'.

Where to Find Alternatives

Organic produce retailers often also supply other products, such as ranges of biodegradable cleaning agents. Your local health food shop will probably have non-chemical cosmetics and toiletries, and so will some chemists, such as Boots.

Other Possible Environmental Pollutants

Of course, it is not just chemicals which can cause allergies. Troublesome particles in the air can be biological as well as chemical. The most common things to be allergic to in this category are:

- dust
- house dust mite
- mould spores
- pollens
- cat and dog dander.

It is important to keep rooms clean and dusted, especially the bedroom.

ECOLOGY IN EVERYDAY LIFE

Apart from avoiding the chemicals listed above, there are many other things you can do in your everyday life to make your environment healthier.

- Do not use aluminium saucepans or frying pans for cooking. If you have any, throw them out. Minute particles of aluminium can get into the food you eat which is cooked in these utensils. This has been associated with conditions such as senile dementia and Alzheimer's disease.
- Eat nothing out of tins. Particles of the tin can seep into the foods and contaminate them. It is always better to eat fresh foods anyway, with frozen as a second best.

The Contraceptive Pill

Dr Ellen Grant, author of *The Bitter Pill* (Corgi, 1986) believes the increasing incidence of MS, especially among young women, can be linked with the pill, which has been in widespread use since the mid 1960s. The pill, amongst its many other actions, robs the body of zinc. Any women with MS would be better off using another form of contraception which does not involve chemicals.

Microwaves from Transmitters

This theory comes from Sheffield scientist Dr Jane G Clarke, who has written a book called *Multiple Sclerosis – A New Theory Concerning Cause and Cure* (New Age Science Press, 1983). Her main thesis is that the damage seen in MS is due to overheating of the myelin sheath. The overheating is brought on by various factors, the most controversial one being microwaves, particularly radar waves in the 10cm waveband, which bypass the skin's heat receptors. Dr Clarke suggests that people who get MS have been brought up on a copper-deficient diet, so their myelin never reaches normal thickness.

More information from:

New Age Science Press Ltd,
66 Hatings Road,
Millhouses,
Sheffield S7 2GU.

Electrical Equipment

Theories about the effects of electrical equipment can be obtained from:

Dr Cyril Smith,
Electrical Engineering Dept,
Salford University,
Manchester.

Vaccinations

The view that vaccinations may be implicated in MS is shared by several holistic practitioners, including the late Dr Robert S Mendelsohn, editor of *The People's Doctor* (PO Box 982, Evanston, Illinois 60204).

Dr Mendelsohn wrote: 'While scientists have spent millions of dollars in a fruitless chase of possible viruses that might cause MS, I believe the most overlooked area of research is that which doctors call iatrogenic (doctor-produced). Since it is highly unlikely that any miracle drug will be found, I would recommend that every MS researcher and all the various fund-raising organizations pursue factors that may prevent MS. High on my list of suspicious doctor-caused factors are delayed reactions to infant formula, routine immunizations, and allergy shots. After all, we now know that another serious neurologic condition, Guillain-Barre paralysis, comes from the swine flu vaccine and other vaccines.' (*The People's Doctor* Vol 6 no 5).

Another alternative practitioner who shares this view is Leon Chaitow, whose book *Vaccination and Immunisation: Dangers, Delusions and Alternatives* (C.W. Daniel) was nominated as book of the year by the *Journal of Alternative Medicine* in the UK in 1989.

Many people with MS report that their first symptoms followed shortly after some vaccination, such as smallpox. This may or may not be coincidental.

It is probably safer to avoid any further vaccinations once MS is diagnosed, even though this might restrict visiting certain countries. If you can stand your ground against doctors, you might also consider saying no to all vaccinations to your children (except those for tetanus and polio).

Carbon Monoxide Pollution

MS is common in those areas of the world where there is carbon monoxide pollution of the air. Carbon monoxide poisoning can lead to the demyelination and degeneration of the central nervous system in laboratory animals. It has been shown that exposure to carbon monoxide increases the need for pyridoxine (B6). A hypothesis has been put forward suggesting that a relative B6 deficiency may cause MS in susceptible people. (Mitchell DA, Schanell EK, *American J. Clinical Nutrition*, August 1973.)

13

Hyperbaric Oxygen Treatment

WHAT IS HYPERBARIC OXYGEN?

Hyperbaric oxygen (HBO) is oxygen at an increased level of pressure. 'Hyper' means increased, 'baric' means pressure. You go into a special chamber with increased atmospheric pressure and breathe oxygen through a mask. Under increased pressure there is a higher concentration of oxygen coming in contact with and saturating tissue and blood. All the cells of the body are bathed in this oxygen.

The special chambers used for hyperbaric oxygen treatment look like big metal capsules. A typical one has six or eight seats with portholes. Each seat is equipped with an oxygen feed to which an oxygen mask is connected. During the treatment (sometimes called a 'dive') you put this oxygen mask over your mouth and nose and breathe pure oxygen.

How Does it Work?

No one knows for sure. One of the most popular theories is that of Dr Philip James of Dundee University. He is a consultant in occupational medicine who specializes in diving. He says that MS may result from fatty blockages in tiny blood vessels. The medical term for this is 'fat globule micro-embolism'.

Dr James believes that fat embolism, blockage of fat globules, is responsible for the damage to blood vessels at the onset of every new MS symptom. The damaged vessels leak toxic substances into the surrounding nerve tissues, damaging the myelin sheaths and producing the scattered scars of multiple sclerosis in the central nervous system. If Dr James' fatty blockage theory is right, HBO treatment works because oxygen, when breathed under pressure, dislodges the fat globules and disperses them.

Interestingly, divers who get 'the bends' when they come up from a deep sea dive too fast suffer from symptoms very similar to MS. Their symptoms are the result of air bubbles in the circulation. Dr James suggests that fat globules in the blood block blood vessels in the nervous system in the same way in multiple sclerosis. However, this theory may be only part of the story.

When Dr Richard Neubauer, a doctor practising hyperbaric oxygen medicine in Florida, gave a talk on HBO to ARMS in 1983, he listed several possible different ways HBO might be working. He was certain that oxygen gets right to the nucleus of cells. In addition to that, it regenerates nerve axons, it has good effects on the body's immune system, it reduces or stops swelling in the central nervous system, it increases microcirculation, and it even improves IQ.

Of course, oxygen is vital for healthy people too. It is necessary to all body tissues, but especially to sensitive nerve tissue. If the oxygen level in the blood of a healthy person drops, the blood vessels in the brain dilate and eventually leak, causing brain swelling due to the build-up of liquid.

In the USA hyperbaric oxygen is commonly used in the treatment of about forty conditions. This long list includes drowning, diving accidents, burns, crash injuries, severed limbs, electrocution, smoke inhalation, and cyanide poisoning.

HBO treatment doesn't produce major changes overnight. Increased oxygenation simply allows the natural mechanisms of repair in the body to take place.

What's the Treatment Like?

Of course, what it feels like to have HBO treatment does differ somewhat from person to person. Even so, there are some broad guidelines.

You are seated in the chamber with other people having the treatment. When everyone is settled, the chamber operators begin the 'descent'. They tell you when to put on your mask and begin breathing oxygen. Most chambers have an intercom system so that the operators can keep you informed about what is happening and you can tell them if there are any problems.

Gradually, the operators increase the pressure inside the chamber. This process can take up to ten minutes, and it's the only

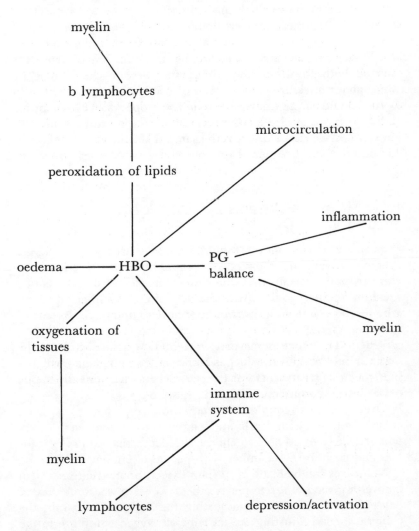

Figure 11: How HBO may be working.

part of the treatment that can be a little bit unpleasant. It's rather like going deep underground in a tube train or taking off in an aeroplane – your ears pop. The trick is to keep swallowing.

Once you're 'down' (you don't go anywhere – it's just that the atmosphere has changed so that it's like being deep under the sea) you stay for about an hour and a half. All you do is sit there, with your mask on, breathing oxygen. Many people like to take along books or magazines to help pass the time.

In some treatment centres, there is a 'half-time', during which you can take off your mask, have a bit of a rest, and breathe normal air. By the way, the air in the chamber at all times feels perfectly normal both to sit in and to breathe, despite the change in atmospheric pressure.

At the end of the treatment period, the operators slowly bring you 'up' to sea level – again taking about ten minutes. Once the pressure inside the chamber is the same as the air outside, the air-locked door can be opened and out you go.

How Many Treatments Do You Need? And At What Depth?

How many treatments you should have, how deep you should go, and exactly how much oxygen you should breathe have not been standardized. It seems that what works for one person may not be ideal for another, so that, with the help of the chamber operators who will be monitoring you, you may have to find the best method for you.

When HBO treatments first started, it was thought that the depth should be 33 feet, which is known as 'two atmospheres'. The best course of treatments was thought to be twenty-one dives, one each day, taken on consecutive days, six days a week.

Over the last couple of years, however, there has been experimentation with depths and lengths of treatment, so that now you are likely to be able to choose the depth that works best for you and go into the chamber with people of similar need.

Now dives can be 8, 10, 16, 24, or 33 feet. Some treatments can be over a period of three weeks, others over five weeks. A dose of oxygen can be altered by adjusting the pressure of air in the chamber or by adjusting the amount of oxygen coming into the mask.

Why Do You Have To Be in a Chamber At All?

People often ask why you can't just breathe oxygen sitting at home in an armchair. The answer is that when you breathe oxygen at normal pressures you cannot reach the same oxygen content in the blood as when you breathe oxygen under increased pressure. Using oxygen at an increased atmospheric pressure reduces the diameter of blood vessels in the nervous system. Despite the reduction in blood-flow, the delivery of oxygen to the tissues is in fact increased. This may sound like a paradox, but it's true.

Top-Ups

From the research done so far, it seems that 'top-ups', or maintenance treatments, are essential to any improvement and keep the disease stable, though how often you have a top-up does vary from person to person. For some people, it could be as often as twice a week, particularly for those people with fluctuating symptoms. For others, whose conditions are more stable, it could be every ten days or longer.

The pressure level in the top-up sessions is usually the same as used in the initial treatment course.

Dr James says that HBO should be thought of as a supplement, a bit like insulin to a diabetic. So top-up treatments should not be neglected, in case old symptoms come back.

Hints During HBO Treatment

1. Eat a nutritious diet (see chapter 3). Have something to eat and drink before you go into the chamber.
2. It can be colder inside the chamber than in the outer room, so wear comfortable, warm clothes. But don't wear anything nylon or other static-prone materials that might create a spark. Take off your watch, as the increased pressure inside the chamber can cause the cover of the watch face to pop off.
3. Give a list of all the drugs and medications you are taking to the operators.
4. Tell them if you have a bad cold, as this can make the ear problems worse. You might be advised to skip a treatment or two until the cold has gone.

5. There are divided views on whether you should be allowed to have sweets or gum, as you might when a plane is taking off or landing. Many people have found that swallowing does lessen the ear problems, but some centres have found that moving the jaw has interfered with the oxygen masks. So you had better ask your centre operator about this.
6. Take in a good book, magazines, crossword puzzles, or whatever will keep you from getting bored. The lighting is bright enough to read.
7. Cigarette smoking is absolutely forbidden either in the chamber or in the centres. Nothing flammable may be taken inside the chamber and no petroleum-based products may be worn on the body.

Does HBO Work?

No one is claiming that HBO is a cure for MS. To be realistic, HBO can't instantly put to rights long-term deterioration. But many people do respond once the right pressure and the right length of treatment have been found. It seems that even the patients who don't improve can sometimes remain stable. So if it achieves nothing else, HBO may be able to stabilize MS.

However, there is no doubt that some people do improve as a result of HBO. Dr Richard Neubauer says, 'The changes are so obvious, an idiot could see them.' Unfortunately, these changes don't happen to everyone.

The most positive research so far comes from Dr Boguslav Fischer and his colleagues at the New York University Medical Center. The study was published in the New England Journal of Medicine in 1982. In the group who were given HBO, there was an immediate improvement in 12 out of 17. In the control group, there was an improvement in only 1 out of 20. After a year, deterioration was noticed in 2 patients in the HBO group and 11 patients in the control group. The good results from the HBO treatment wore off in 7 of the treated group, but were long-lasting in 5.

Dr Fischer himself is quoted as saying that HBO produces 'a possible slowing of the progression of the disease'. But he concluded that more research is needed. 'This therapy cannot be generally recommended without longer follow-up periods and additional confirmatory experience.'

A leading place for HBO in the UK is Dundee, largely because Dr Philip James is at Dundee University, and also because ARMS has a particularly active HBO centre there, which was the first in the UK.

In 1983 a pilot study was conducted by Dr Duncan Davison of Dundee for ARMS, though this was not a controlled trial. The results were not wonderful, but not bad. Out of 38 patients (11 male, 27 female) a third reported improvements in bladder function, sensation and muscle co-ordination in the three weeks following HBO treatment. These people did not improve in other MS symptoms.

Thirteen patients described feeling better during treatment, and this improvement started at any time between the first treatment and the seventeenth treatment. One patient described herself as feeling mentally hyperactive for several hours after each session.

On the Disability Status Scale (a measure for physical disability), 4 patients improved by 1 point and were considered to be moderately improved.

Some patients noted differences in their motor function which made a significant difference in their daily life. Four patients described an important increase in the distance they could walk before they got fatigued. For example, a person who used to be able to walk only 300 yards before HBO treatment could walk a mile after it. However, in two of these patients there was deterioration within seven days of the end of the treatment. In one of them the deterioration was so significant that he was worse than before the treatment started.

These are some of the remarks made by the patients who noticed improvement in their motor functions, such as walking and moving their arms. 'Less trailing of the legs when walking'; 'less footdrop in the right leg'; 'increased power in the hand'; 'slight increase in power'; 'writing better'.

A third of the patients noted an improvement in what neurologists call 'cerebellar function' – nodding the head, shakiness, unsteadiness. The improvements were less shakiness and the ability to stand on a chair or to stand up without feeling unsteady. No patient had a dramatic improvement in 'cerebellar function' and two got worse.

Fourteen patients improved sensory functions – 44 per cent of the total. These people noted: loss of the 'bandaged' feeling under the chest; return of feeling to hands or fingers; lessening of pain in the limbs. On the other hand, 5 patients went the other way and suffered loss of sensation, more pain, more tingling, and more numbness. As compared to the 44 per cent who improved, 3 per cent worsened.

In bowel and bladder functions, there was improvement in 10 patients, or 37 per cent. No patient got worse in bladder function. There was no significant change in bowel function. In the group in which bladder function improved, one said that he used to have to go to the toilet every hour before the HBO, but after the HBO he only needed to go once every four to five hours; another said she used to have to get up two or three times in the night and now she had to get up only once or not at all; another said her visits to the toilet had reduced from once every one to one and half hours, to once every two or three hours, with less urgency too. There is no doubt from the Davison study that the clearest benefits were in bladder symptoms.

Dr Davison's conclusion was:

> Improvements in approximately one third of patients with bladder symptoms, sensory symptoms and ataxia were described, but no benefit overall in other functions. The changes appear to be greater than may be anticipated from the placebo response, suggesting that hyperbaric oxygen does have an effect on the nervous system.

However, striking results have been reported by Dr Neubauer in the USA. In one study (1980) of 250 patients with MS, he reported a 'dramatic' improvement in 39 per cent, minimal and moderate improvement in 52 per cent, and no improvement in 9 per cent. He reported similar results in another study (1982) of 600 patients, where the experience of his own unit was pooled with patients being treated in Houston, Texas, and in Naples, Italy.

Research on HBO

However, research in the period 1982–1986 was not able to repeat the good results of Fischer and Neubauer in the USA. Indeed, research trials on HBO have found there is no significant benefit *overall* in MS with HBO treatment.

Two major trials in the UK were commissioned by the MS

Society of Great Britain and N. Ireland, one in Newcastle, and the other at St Thomas's Hospital and Whipps Cross Hospital in London. The Newcastle results were published in *The Lancet* in February 1985; the London results in the *British Medical Journal* in February 1986. Both trials could find no significant benefit of HBO on overall MS symptoms. However, the Newcastle trial did find there was a small but significant subjective improvement in bladder function.

The London study of 84 patients could find no clinically important or significant benefit in either the patient's subjective opinion, the examiner's opinion, the score on the Kurtzke disability status scale (see page 55), or the time taken to walk 50 metres.

All the doctors involved in these major trials reached the same conclusion – that HBO is not an effective treatment for MS.

The authors of the paper published in the *British Medical Journal* conclude:

> The results . . . on a total of 204 patients studied under double blind conditions in the United Kingdom fit in with the findings of several smaller studies recently reported in the USA . . . our findings, obtained with detailed methods of assessment . . . have failed to confirm those of Fischer *et al*. There appears to be little basis for recommending this treatment to patients with multiple sclerosis.

David Bates, Professor of Neurology at the Royal Victoria Infirmary in Newcastle was one of the doctors on the Newcastle study. He feels that the negative result from these two major studies should refute once and for all the suggestion that HBO should be part of the management of MS.

But despite these trials, the controversy still continues. Those who support HBO still do so, challenging those doctors who feel they have proved it is ineffective.

One of the main supporters of HBO is Dr Philip James of Dundee. He criticizes the Newcastle and London trials on various scores. Firstly, the patients were treated at 2 atmospheres absolute, which may be too much; secondly, the patients in the trials were not given top-ups, which he considers very important; thirdly, he thinks that the patients selected for the trials should not have been chronic cases. He argues that HBO may be best suited for *acute* cases of MS.

The other therapeutic uses for HBO do use it for acute circumstances. Dr James feels it is indefensible to wait for a patient to get worse – to the point where the condition is irreversible – before starting treatment.

As in all therapies, Dr James claims that it works best for those patients who are not yet badly disabled.

However, in answer to Dr James's criticisms, the doctors involved in the two big UK trials say that they followed very closely the protocol of the Fischer study in the USA, which had such favourable results.

However, the poor results of HBO for MS as reported from Newcastle and London do not tally with other results, particularly from Italy.

Professor Damiano Zannini, and others, from the Hyperbaric Medicine Center in Genoa, Italy, found that HBO is beneficial for MS patients.

He concluded that:

• Improvements or regression or symptoms, or functional recovery, can be observed.
• These improvements can be lasting or temporary.
• A trend towards the disease worsening was halted.
• The symptoms most likely to improve were cerebellar (e.g. shakiness, unsteadiness, head nodding), sensory, and sphincteric (bladder and bowel control).

But he did feel that HBO was still an experimental treatment, until further research was done.

Bladder and Bowel Control

What seems to be emerging from various trials is that the symptoms which HBO helps most are bladder and bowel control.

Even the Bates trial in Newcastle, which found no *overall* benefit of HBO, did find it helped bladder and bowel symptoms – 12 out of 51 patients in the HBO group, compared with only 3 out of the 47 control patients, felt the HBO had helped their bladder and bowel symptoms.

Other studies done in various parts of the world back up these results – 25–50 per cent of patients on HBO report improvement in bladder and bowel function. Dr Appell in Louisiana and Dr Neubauer in Florida draw particular attention to improvements in bladder and bowel function.

This improvement in bladder function was somewhat glossed over by the Newcastle doctors in their report in *The Lancet*. This is challenged by Dr Philip James:

> Objective evidence of improvement in bladder function with hyperbaric oxygen therapy has been produced by urologists under double-blind conditions. It is clearly wrong to discount the importance of bladder function in the management of patients with chronic multiple sclerosis, in view of the associated morbidity and the effects of bladder dysfunction on the quality of life.

'Subjective' Results – The ARMS Study

Normally, patients in medical trials are assessed objectively by specialists, and 'subjective' assessments tend not to be taken into consideration (although they were considered in the trial done at St Thomas's and Whipps Cross Hospitals).

ARMS decided to look at HBO from the patient's subjective point of view, i.e. how they themselves felt about the treatment. Fifty participants filled in questionnaires which covered much wider aspects of health than is usually covered. The questions included areas of personal and social life, as well as physical and psychological health.

The participants in this trial were divided into two groups, A and B. Each group had an 8-week regime of HBO plus top-ups (regime 1) then crossed over to an 8-week regime of air plus top-ups (regime 2). This is called a double blind, controlled, crossover trial. In all, the participants had 20 treatments of HBO plus top-ups, and 16 treatments of air.

The conclusion was that, although there was little evidence of improvement related specifically to HBO, most participants did report effects which they themselves attributed to HBO.

Participants from different social backgrounds responded differently to the trial.

There were significant changes for the better reported in relation to sleeping better, having more energy, feeling less socially isolated, and having a more rewarding social life.

On specific MS symptoms, the majority felt they had improved. Increased mobility and improved urinary symptoms were the two areas which people said had improved most.

There is a very big difference between the HBO therapy given at ARMS centres around the country and the HBO treatment given as part of the Newcastle and London trials. Going to the HBO chamber in an ARMS centre is a social event. You meet people and make friends. You share the experience in a multi-chamber with several other people. The chamber becomes a friendly place, a place where people can tell jokes, play card games, natter, or just read.

In the big trials, the HBO was just a treatment. Indeed, at St Thomas's and Whipp's Cross Hospitals, the HBO was in single, one-person chambers, so there was no chance of any sociability attached to the therapy.

Perhaps one of the therapeutic aspects of the kind of HBO given at ARMS centres is that it is like a club; people's spirits are raised and they feel better – both mentally and physically.

ARMS HBO Centres – Anecdotal Reports

The results of recent scientific trials into HBO have not been good. But you could visit any ARMS HBO centre anywhere in the country and hear stories of people making dramatic improvements. There are anecdotes of people who went into the chamber in a wheelchair and came out walking.

On the other hand, you would also hear stories of people gaining no improvement whatsoever.

Most stories would relate minor improvements, such as being able to hold a cup without shaking, or longer intervals between visits to the toilet. This sort of mild improvement in activities of daily living would not feature in the results of a big scientific trial, where one needs to move up a point on the Disability Scale before improvements are considered significant. Yet for someone to be able to hold a cup without spilling its content *is* a major improvement in their daily quality of life.

No one is claiming HBO is a cure for MS. But – despite the trial results – it may help stabilize or improve some symptoms of MS. The less disabled you are, the greater the chance of HBO being of benefit.

The ARMS position as of February 1989 is as follows:

'Hyperbaric Oxygen Therapy (HBO) is *not* a cure for MS – but it does seem effective in helping many people with MS to avoid getting worse. In addition, it often succeeds in obtaining some improvement in the general condition.

The most significant benefits are in improved balance, sensory perception, and control of incontinence. Other symptoms also show beneficial change in different people.

In the period 1938–1987, ARMS Therapy Centres provided 500,000 individual sessions. Around half of the 4,000 people involved have benefited in one or more ways.'

Neurological Benefits in the ARMS Trial

Dr Alec Forti, the neurologist at the ARMS Unit at the Central Middlesex Hospital, made some interesting analyses from the ARMS trial. He concluded that there were no large benefits from HBO if you took the groups studied as a whole. But once you broke down the big groups into sub-groups, there were some benefits. The most significant improvements were in eye/hand co-ordination, and peak flow.

SHOULD HBO BE GIVEN TO EARLY CASES AND ACUTE CASES OF MS?

Again, if the results of trials are analysed in a different way, the picture that emerges is that the recently diagnosed and those with a slower course of the disease without any irreversible disability show the highest percentage of improvement from HBO therapy. Professor Pallotta, from Naples, Italy, followed 100 MS patients between 1977 and 1981, on HBO therapy. He concluded: 'the clinical case with a slower course and those recently diagnosed showed the highest percentage of improvement'.

Dr Philip James, in a letter sent to the *British Medical Journal* in February 1986, argues very strongly for early treatment with HBO. He is very angry that only chronically disabled patients were selected for the big trials on HBO.

He writes: 'The wisdom in choosing chronically disabled patients in trials of therapy in multiple sclerosis, or indeed for trials of therapy in any disease, must be challenged.'

Dr James says that symptoms present for a short time are much more likely to remit given oxygen therapy than long-term problems.

Rather than wait for a patient to be incurably scarred before even making a diagnosis, Dr James urges that doctors refer patients for HBO therapy as soon as someone suffers an acute attack.

He feels that if patients suffering acute attacks were given immediate HBO, it would offer the hope of preventing further disability.

Yet MS people who had recently suffered an acute attack were excluded from the big trials.

Dr James is very critical of those of the medical establishment who sit back and allow an acute condition to turn into a chronic condition. He says: 'We need to remove the ridiculous and self-defeating requirements for multiple lesions to be present before trials of therapy can be undertaken.'

IS HBO SAFE?

In all the fuss in Britain about HBO, there have been some press reports suggesting that MS people could be 'burnt alive' in pressurized oxygen chambers. This is nonsense. It is true that certain hyperbaric oxygen chambers used in hospitals don't use oxygen masks but fill the whole chamber with oxygen. In this situation, a spark could ignite with disastrous results. But the HBO chambers as used by local ARMS groups are not like that. The chambers are filled with ordinary room air. The only pure oxygen is from the masks, and basic precautions are taken to eliminate any possibility of a spark. In addition, both the UK and US governments inspect pressure vessels and approve them for human occupancy.

The other issue over which there is some controversy is whether there should be professional technicians operating the chambers. In fact the chambers are quite easy to operate. The ARMS centres in the UK have many volunteers, most of whom are family or friends of someone with MS. As operators of the chambers they are especially involved, concerned, and caring people.

However, some experts feel that it is essential to have trained technicians operating the chambers. In the US an accredited course is currently being developed to train qualified HBO operators. US authorities also stress that treatments should be taken on the recommendation and under the jurisdiction of a physician.

Does HBO Have Side-Effects?

Probably the most common side-effect is ear-popping. In some people, this can be worse than the sensation you get in your ears when a plane takes off or lands. But this side-effect is lessened if the operator alters the pressure in the chamber very slowly going down and coming up again. The operators normally hold the chamber at a certain pressure level for a little while before going on to the next. This allows the people inside the chamber to get used to each pressure level.

The other common side-effect is on the eyes. The oxygen affects the lens of the eye so that for a short time you may not be able to see as well as normal. But this side-effect usually disappears within an hour or so after each treatment.

Sleepiness is the other frequently-mentioned side-effect. However, it has been found that this sleepiness often indicates that improvement is taking place. This terrible tiredness tends to affect different people at different stages of the treatment. For some, it can happen during the first week; for others, the last week.

Because tiredness is so common for the first week or so of the treatment, it's important to plan absolutely nothing which could tire you during the HBO course. And it would be sensible to ask someone else to drive you home, because your vision may not be up to it for an hour or so after the treatment.

However, once the tiredness phase has passed, people frequently report a feeling of extra energy and liveliness. Some people experience the 'high' of oxygen, in which you feel elated or euphoric. Unfortunately, this pleasant side-effect doesn't last.

Another thing that can happen is that, when you do get sensations back, ironically, they might actually feel bad. For example, when an area of numb skin gets its sensation back, you may feel 'pins and needles'.

In the Dundee study, apart from the ear problems, two patients said they had a bigger appetite; one lost appetite and thirteen pounds in weight. Two patients complained of vertigo and lightheadedness as a result of HBO. One patient developed migraine attacks during some treatments. Fatigue was said to increase in 9 patients and decrease in 9 patients.

The London study, reported in February 1986 in the *British Medical Journal*, found that unwanted side-effects were quite common in both the group given HBO, and the group given just air. Minor ear discomfort was the commonest problem. But no patient had long-lasting side-effects to their ears. Visual disturbances consisted of blurring of vision, usually towards the end of the treatment, which lasted 30 minutes to six hours after treatment, but for several days in one case. One patient remarked on a disturbance of colour vision after HBO treatment. Two patients became anxious and claustrophobic and had to withdraw from treatment. After ear problems, fatigue was the commonest side-effect.

Anti-Oxidants

Some doctors feel it is important to take anti-oxidants – vitamins E and C in particular – when undergoing HBO treatment. This lessens the risk of free radicals (see page 96).

A total of 84 patients took part in the trials.

	HBO Group	Placebo Group
Ear discomfort	26 (3 severe)	10
Deafness	8	3
Sinus pain	2	1
Headache	4	4
Leg pain	5	4
Visual disturbance	8	3
Nausea	3	1
Fatigue	16	20
Fear or anxiety	9 (2 severe)	5

Table 3: Unwanted Effects of HBO, St Thomas's Hospital and Whipps Cross Hospital Trials.

There are several MS Therapy Centres around the UK offering HBO. For details, see Useful Addresses chapter.

14

Physiotherapy and Exercise

Many MS people are more disabled than they need be. It is *not* part of the disease process of MS to have backs bent forward, arms or legs stuck in unnatural positions (contractures), or atrophied leg muscles. These things only develop because of repeated misuse, and inactivity.

One of the many scandals with MS is that doctors do not refer their patients to physiotherapists early enough, or in anything but an *ad hoc* way. Nor do they usually suggest that activity is much better than inactivity.

Even if a doctor does diagnose MS, he is much more likely to say, 'Just go away and forget about it' than to say that physiotherapy and exercise can help.

Patients with MS who are referred to physiotherapists are mostly referred too late. It is much easier to maintain existing use of limbs, than to try and regain the use of limbs which have become disabled.

Once again, it is a case of shutting the stable door after the horse has bolted. How much saner it would be if people with MS could receive all possible treatments very early on in the disease, before the rot has set in.

Studies have now proved that certain treatments *are* effective and should be started as early in the disease as possible. Physiotherapy/exercise is one of the therapies which has been shown to have real benefits.

WHY PHYSIOTHERAPY/EXERCISE IS SO IMPORTANT

- It improves circulation and all bodily functions.
- It increases the amount of oxygen in the blood.
- It keeps muscles strong and strengthens weak ones.
- It keeps joints mobile and prevents stiffness.
- It may help reduce spasticity.
- It helps maintain maximum independence.
- It lifts depression.
- It gives a feeling of well-being by toning up the whole system.
- It prevents muscles from atrophying.
- It means you can do everyday things better.
- It gives you more energy.
- It helps you look good.
- It helps keep at bay disabilities which are not part of the MS disease process.

If You Don't Use It, You Lose It

Our motto should be, 'If you don't use it, you lose it'. Another good one is 'make the best of what you've got'.

Many of the complications of MS arise from disuse. Contractures, deformities and reduced mobility are often simply put down to being part of having MS. But they are *not* necessarily part of the disease process at all. They come about because of misuse and disuse.

Inactivity can lead to complications. On the other hand, activity can prevent them, or at least delay them.

Regular exercising can make the difference between being able to stand and to walk – or becoming wheelchair-bound.

Fatigue

You may think that you haven't got the energy to do any sort of exercise, and fear that it would make you feel drained.

But the ironic thing about exercise is that it energizes you. Of course, you shouldn't exert yourself so much you're exhausted. But no exercise at all will leave you more fatigued than gentle exercise which keeps the body in good tone.

Exercises are designed not only to increase fitness, but also to increase stamina and endurance. This will take time to build up, but will make you fatigue less easily.

You will learn your own limits of endurance. Stop before you get fatigued, or it could have detrimental effects. Keep cool while exercising to stave off fatigue caused by heat.

Any gross lack of regular exercise causes disuse atrophy. Research has shown that muscle disuse due to immobility results in the selective atrophy of the slow, oxidative, fatigue-resistant type I muscle fibre, as opposed to the fast fatiguing, glucolytic type II fibres.

However, regular exercise changes the biochemical properties of skeletal muscles. Endurance training in particular partially converts the type II fibres from an anaerobic to an aerobic metabolism, making them more fatigue resistant – or more like type I fibres.

EXERCISE YOU CAN DO ON YOUR OWN

If you are active enough to do exercises on your own, you may not need to see a physiotherapist. You can do on your own whatever exercise you enjoy doing most. This might include:

- Walking
- Swimming
- Dancing
- Exercise classes, including stretching and gentle aerobics.
- 'Toning' tables, which help by doing most of the work for you.
- Rebounder exercises.

A rebounder, which looks like a mini trampoline, is very good for building up strength in your leg muscles, and for stamina. If you have a problem with balance, you can put the rebounder near a wall so you can touch the wall to keep your balance. You will be amazed how quickly your jumping ability increases, just by using the rebounder for a couple of minutes every day.

Whatever exercise you choose, do it regularly, ideally every day. It will make a real, noticeable difference to your strength and stamina.

Always stop exercising before you get tired. Never allow yourself to get fatigued.

WHY YOU SHOULD SEE A PHYSIOTHERAPIST EARLY ON

If you see a physiotherapist early on, she or he will be able to prevent secondary handicap – the sort of handicap which is not part of MS but a preventable complication of it. She will help you keep your present abilities, or even to improve on them.

A physiotherapist will design a tailor-made set of exercises just for you, which you can then do on your own, ideally every day.

Ideally, a physiotherapist, or physiotherapists, should continue their involvement with you, taking into account the fluctuations of the disease. At present, patients are rarely referred to a physiotherapist at all, or perhaps only as part of a stay in hospital. If no one suggests it, ask your doctor to refer you to a physiotherapist at your local hospital.

If your particular problems could be identified early on, the physiotherapist could work with you on those problems, and hopefully stop them from developing into something worse. Her aim would be to work out a programme so you could maintain or improve on your present abilities – all your movements, and all your activities of daily living. Physiotherapists talk about 'maintaining a level of function'.

A Partnership Between Patient and Physiotherapist

In a good partnership between a patient and a physiotherapist, the patient is not just passively on the receiving end of treatment, but is actively involved and responsible. This means seeing the management of multiple sclerosis as a way of life, rather than just a series of therapies. It also means understanding the benefits of rest, as well as the benefits of activity. It also means not being lazy, and doing the exercises designed for you.

A physiotherapist will teach you how to stand properly, how to balance properly, how to stand up from sitting and lying, how to walk properly, how to position yourself to sleep, and how to co-ordinate your movements better. He or she will help you be aware of your posture, your movements, and your sensory perception.

There is a right way and a wrong way of doing all those things, and a physiotherapist will teach you the right way to stop you getting into bad habits. Their aim is to bring your body back into balance so you can move more normally and freely and enjoy an active life as long as possible.

POSTURE, SECONDARY HANDICAP, AND EXERCISE

A poor posture may be the first signs of muscle imbalance. It may be hard to stand up properly because of damage to neural mechanisms. But, it is very important to take steps to correct bad posture as it can have knock-on effects: apart from throwing the body out of balance it also has a bad effect on breathing, and also on the internal organs, which will make constipation and incontinence worse than need be. A slouched posture also can cause pains in the neck and shoulders, depression, and flabby muscles. In time, postural abnormalities will have an effect on movement. All the above are examples of secondary handicap which can be avoided.

The best way to prevent postural abnormalities from becoming fixed is a regular, daily stretching routine. A physiotherapist will give you some simple stretching exercises for you to do every day at home. These stretching exercises will stimulate good posture and good balance. Yoga is also very good for correcting postural faults (see chapter 15).

Balance

The loss of balance typical of MS may be due to abnormalities in the inner ear caused by the disease itself. But walking as if you're falling off a tightrope could also be because of very bad posture. You are literally thrown off balance because your body is out of alignment, and the centre of gravity simply falls outside the base of support. To get yourself centred again, the physiotherapist will suggest activities and exercises which stimulate balance. Yoga is also very good for this.

Muscle Tone

One of the things a physiotherapist will identify is abnormalities in muscle tone, as they can create problems with movement. As with bad balance, poor muscle tone can be a secondary effect of

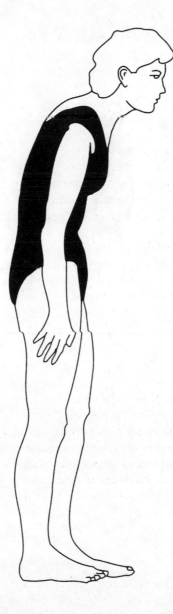

Figure 12: Poor Posture

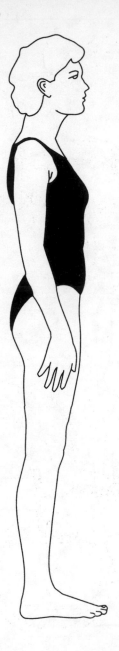

Figure 13: Good Posture

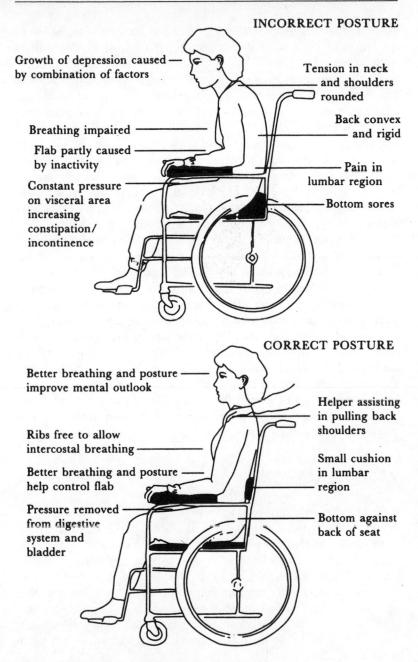

INCORRECT POSTURE

Growth of depression caused by combination of factors

Tension in neck and shoulders rounded

Breathing impaired

Back convex and rigid

Flab partly caused by inactivity

Constant pressure on visceral area increasing constipation/ incontinence

Pain in lumbar region

Bottom sores

CORRECT POSTURE

Better breathing and posture improve mental outlook

Helper assisting in pulling back shoulders

Ribs free to allow intercostal breathing

Small cushion in lumbar region

Better breathing and posture help control flab

Pressure removed from digestive system and bladder

Bottom against back of seat

Figure 14: Good and bad posture in a wheelchair

poor posture. In people suffering from MS, muscles can be either flaccid, with no tone; or the opposite, spastic; or else atrophied from disuse.

If the muscles have too much tone, i.e. are spastic, the physiotherapist will design a programme which avoids positions and activities which increase tone, or which reinforce abnormal ways of moving. The programme will include daily walking or standing, also weight-bearing and regular stretching. She will also advise on how to avoid pressure sores, constipation and bladder infections.

One of the things that is *not* helpful is to increase the strength of muscles that are strong already. This only makes the weaker ones weaker. If, for example, you are strong from the waist upwards, but weak from the waist downwards, there is the temptation to use your arms and trunk a lot, not your legs and lower half.

There is a theory about 'associated reactions' which goes like this: the more you use your right hand, the weaker your left hand gets; the more you use your arms, the weaker your legs get; one part of your body may well be compensating for another part.

Concentrate on the weak areas; the strong areas can take care of themselves. That way you have the chance of bringing your body back into balance. If you only build up the strong muscles, so that the weak ones stand no chance, the more out of balance you will be. That is why you should be careful not to put your weight on your hands when you sit down or get up from an armchair. Use your legs as much as you can.

WHAT EXERCISES?

If you see a physiotherapist, she will design a set of exercises tailor-made to your particular needs and disability. Gentle stretching exercises are likely to be part of this. Such exercises will be designed to make the most of what you've got, correct any postural faults, get you back on balance, and rectify abnormal muscle tone.

There is also nothing to stop you doing any kind of exercise that appeals to you. Obviously, what exercise you do depends on how disabled you are. Some people who have MS can play squash; others are grateful to be able to touch their toes while sitting in their wheelchair.

If you are unable to move easily, there is no reason why you should not join any ordinary gym in your local area. Tell the instructor that you have MS so you will not be forced to do things beyond your ability or stamina, and so that you can rest when you feel like it.

Any form of exercise will do you good. It does not have to be a formal class. If you have the self-discipline, you could exercise at home. But whatever you do, do it regularly; ideally, every day.

Swimming is the best form of exercise there is, and ideal for disabled people as long as the water is warmer than in normal pools. Enquire whether there are any special swimming pools, or swimming sessions, in your area.

Various MS groups around the country offer their own physiotherapy and exercise sessions.

Some branches of the MS Society have exercise groups combining exercise and physiotherapy with advice on diet and also counselling. You can get a list of these centres by writing to:

Multiple Sclerosis Society of Great Britain
   and Northern Ireland
25 Effie Road
London SW6 1EE
Tel: 0171-610 7171

Helplines: London 0171-222 3123 (24 hours)
           Midlands 0121-476 4229
           Scotland 0131-226 6573

RESEARCH IN PHYSIOTHERAPY

The physiotherapists at the MS Unit at the Central Middlesex Hospital conducted a retrospective study to find out whether physiotherapy had any beneficial effects on the symptoms of MS.

The results were very clear: the patients who had the most physiotherapy – averaging 8 hours per month – did best. And the ones who had least physiotherapy – averaging half an hour a month – did worst.

The physiotherapists did assessments of the patients in these areas: the voluntary control of a range of lower limb movements; activities such as getting in and out of bed, in and out of chairs, etc.; balance activities; and activities of daily living.

In all, 40 patients took part in this study. All of these had been attending for physiotherapy at the ARMS Unit for longer than a year. They all had a definite diagnosis of MS; none had suffered a relapse over a period of 18 months; all of them had some problems with movement; and none of them suffered from any other condition that would have complicated the picture.

The patients were assessed every 6 months over an 18-month period.

One of the observations of the physiotherapists was that the patient's general condition got steadily worse, even though they did not suffer actual relapses. Changes in the group of 40 showed that there was a highly significant progression towards greater disability with a loss of range in voluntary movements in the lower limbs.

On the other hand, the patients generally stayed the same in functional and also in balance activities. And in activities of daily living, there were some real improvements towards more independence. The greatest changes were made in the first six months.

At one point the physiotherapists changed the emphasis of the treatment to include more functional activities. At another point the emphasis was switched to balance activities. Once the accent was taken away from functional activities, these got worse. This showed that the content of the physiotherapy made a difference.

Not surprisingly, the physiotherapists found that if someone improved in one area, it was likely to have a good effect on other areas.

Attenders Did Much Better than Non-Attenders

Looking back over the 18-month period of the study, the physiotherapists were able to see that it was possible to rank the 40 participants in order of how much and how little physiotherapy they had received.

Group A consisted of the 14 MS patients who had received the most physiotherapy. Group B consisted of the 14 patients who had received the least physiotherapy. Both groups were comparable in terms of where they stood on the Kurtzke disability scale at the start of the study.

The results were very encouraging. Although both groups did

deteriorate in their range of voluntary movements, group A, who had received the most physiotherapy, deteriorated significantly less than group B, who had received the least physiotherapy.

Physiotherapy did not actually prevent deterioration in voluntary range of movements, but it did slow it down. There were also significant differences between the two groups in balance activities, and activities of daily living. The group who had the most physiotherapy got the most benefit. In activities of daily living, they actually improved their abilities. In functional activities, where there was no marked difference between the two groups, group A still fared better than group B.

Why the Physiotherapy Worked

Postural abnormalities were corrected; abnormal movements were corrected; patients learned or re-learned new strategies of movement. The regular exercise maximized the potential of the muscles and meant that the muscles did not stop working, did not stop being used, and so did not atrophy.

Conclusions from the ARMS Physiotherapy Study

1. Disability caused by postural deformity or disuse atrophy can be minimized.
2. Several movement abnormalities can be prevented or delayed.
3. Abilities can be maximized.
4. The patients who get the most out of physiotherapy are those who:
   - are referred early
   - have regular assessments
   - have long-term treatment
   - have regular treatment.
5. Without early referral, regular assessments, long-term treatment or regular treatment, patients' disabilities get worse. These disabilities are secondary handicap, caused by misuse and disuse, and are not part of the disease process itself.

It's worth repeating – regular exercise can make the difference between the patient retaining his ability to stand or walk – or becoming wheelchair-bound.

Neuromuscular Stimulation (NMS)

Neuromuscular stimulation is a recent technique. A low frequency muscle stimulator makes the lower limb muscles contract, using an electrical impulse. Patients are asked to contract the muscle voluntarily to coincide with the stimulation cycle.

Clinical studies have shown a measurable improvement in the range of lower limb movements, and in walking rate which reversed a previous trend towards slow deterioration. NMS must be done under the supervision of a physiotherapist.

EXERCISES TO HELP MS

Good exercises for MS include stretching, swimming and weight training. You can also do any sport you enjoy within your capabilities.

Exercises specifically designed to help MS, based on Conductive Education from the Peto Institute in Hungary, have been developed in the UK and are available in Chelmsford and Birmingham. This type of exercise helps improve mobility, developing new skills to help sufferers make the most of their abilities and lead more active and independent lives. Conductive Education teachers believe that if you don't use it, you lose it. They use resistance exercises, rather than aerobics, to help strengthen the immune system.

You can learn to do many simple exercises, such as calf muscle lifts and stretches, at home every day. It is important to do a type of exercise that suits you, and which does not cause fatigue.

Exercise in cool conditions, rest when you need to, and never overdo it – always stop before you overheat or get tired.

Where to Go

Many people with MS simply go to their local gym or swimming pool. Some MS Society branches and MS Therapy Centres include exercise. Passive exercises are useful for people who cannot do active exercising and there are many good products available. Look for ads in *MS Matters*.

The following places have exercises and equipment specially designed for people with MS:

National Institute of Conductive Education
Cannon Hill House
Russell Road
Moseley
Birmingham B13 8RD
Tel: 0121-449 1569

A clinic run by Susie Cornell, who has MS, uses resistance exercises against weights, together with reflexology, massage, diet advice and nutritional supplements.

Under Pressure
Navigation Road
Chelmsford
Essex CM2 6HE
Tel: 01245 268098

15

Yoga

Yoga deserves a chapter to itself, separate from the exercise chapter, because it is more a total philosophy than a simple set of postures or keep-fit exercises. It has as much to do with your whole attitude to life, and the way you breathe, as about postures.

Yoga is a unity of the mental and the physical. Done properly, it calms the mind and energizes the body. The body and mind are bound up together and cannot be separated. With a strong sense of purpose, the mind can have a powerful influence on the body.

Hatha yoga is based on the system of the relationship between mind and body. It concentrates on the whole body, so as well as developing physical health, it also promotes mental health.

The word 'Yoga' comes from the Sanskrit and means 'join' or 'unite'. Hatha yoga is about reaching a balance between the positive and negative within oneself. (Ha – sun: positive; tha – moon: negative.)

YOGA AND DIS-EASE

The yogic philosophy is that good health is the natural state for human beings. Good health is when the body and mind are in a state of equilibrium. Illness, or dis-ease, is when the body and mind are out of balance.

There is a natural life force within us all that is trying to do its best to keep us healthy. Yogis say that one does not become ill if one leads a natural life. Even if you have been leading the unhealthy lifestyle of western civilization, the body's healing powers are still there, just waiting to be given a fair chance.

YOGA AND MULTIPLE SCLEROSIS

Since the late 1970s, many people with MS have been doing yoga. The Yoga for Health Foundation in Bedfordshire has done a great deal of work with MS people, and it has proved of great benefit.

Howard Kent, the director of the Yoga for Health Foundation says: 'We have evidence that where people are effectively maintaining yoga both mentally and physically, it is rare for us to find deterioration.'

In an anecdotal way, you will frequently find that someone with MS has become a real devotee of yoga, thanks to the benefits they have experienced from it.

Yoga has many advantages for someone with MS:

• Yoga may help the body's own self-healing mechanism and may slow down or even halt the disease process.
• Yoga stills the mind.
• Yoga increases energy and counteracts fatigue.
• Yoga lifts the mood and counteracts depression.
• Yoga has a good effect on the functioning of the endocrine glands, the circulatory and respiratory systems, and improves well-being.
• Yoga does not need any special equipment and you can practise it daily at home.

Every Breath You Take, Every Move You Make

Correct breathing is one of the most important aspects of yoga. You may think that breathing is something that everyone does naturally. But in fact 99 per cent of the population breathes incorrectly, with correspondingly ill effects on their bodies.

Breathing is the most important biological function of the body. Every other activity of the body is closely connected with breathing. To realize just how important breathing is, remember that you could live for weeks without food, days without water, but only a few minutes without air. Breathing is of primary importance to one's state of health, emotional outlook, and length of life.

Most people in the West take short rapid shallow breaths, but it is the deep, rhythmic breathing which brings health and energy.

Any shock makes people seize up. Notice how you breathe out with a sigh of relief when some ordeal is over. When people are anxious, they tend not to breathe out enough. 'I held my breath' is a common phrase for being excited or nervous about something. Yet, if you hold your breath often enough, or only breathe in a shallow way, your body is not going to get the oxygen it needs for energy.

If the energy is not flowing properly, it will affect both your body and your brain. You will get fatigued easily, feel run down, and depressed. If you are breathing deeply and rhythmically, you will find it hard to be tense at the same time.

Breath is the source of energy. Life is breath.

All forms of mental un-ease or physical dis-ease give themselves away in the way you breathe. Someone with MS may well be breathing incorrectly because of the mental and physical difficulties brought on by the disease. This creates a vicious circle, because the breathing difficulties themselves only make those problems worse. The way to stop the vicious circle is to exercise control over your breathing. Fortunately, how you breathe is under your voluntary control.

Yoga is about deep abdominal breathing. In a yoga class, you would be taught to be aware of your diaphragm, and to breathe down your abdomen instead of up in your chest. You would learn the essentials of breathing, about the breath of relaxation and the breath of energization. Correct breathing is the foundation on which the other aspects of yoga are based.

The best place to learn correct breathing is in a yoga class, under the supervision of a good teacher.

The importance of correct breathing is summed up by Howard Kent:

> Effective health, mental and physical, depends upon the ability to breathe naturally in an energizing manner and then, when necessity demands it, to breathe in a relaxed way. Many people can do neither and their lives are then largely led in limbo. As a result, effective opposition to any illness or disability proves impossible and deterioration has to set in. That may sound to be a dogmatic statement, but it is true and identifiable.

Stress and Tension

One of the Catch 22s of MS is that stress and tension probably play some part in bringing on an attack of MS; but once you have MS, this in itself creates stress and tension both physically and mentally.

The tension created by having MS can seize up the solar plexus (the network of nerves behind the stomach). This interferes with the movement of the diaphragm, and the body's energy flow is blocked. Yoga relaxes the body, opens up the diaphragm, and frees the energy flow.

Problems with balance and movement will make your body try and compensate by using other muscles. This can create unnatural muscle tensions, which, if they go on for a long time, will lead to spasticity and also affect the functioning of the area around the tense muscles. Once your postural abnormalities have been corrected, and you have learned how to relax through correct deep breathing, your body will be able to move more freely.

One of the causes of tension in MS is a profound feeling of self-consciousness about your disabled body. Once you lose this incapacitating self-consciousness, you would be surprised how much the condition improved once you relaxed. Spasms, spasticity, and clumsiness are worse when you are anxious and self-conscious. If you don't think about it, and can relax, these symptoms are far less pronounced.

The practice of yoga can help alleviate both the physical and mental stresses and tensions.

A Peaceful Mind

Most people's minds are forever buzzing with trivial things. One of the most difficult things to do in yoga is to clear your mind. The rubbish piles up in your mind and races through your head. Yoga aims to clear the debris from your mind. 'Yoga is controlling the activities of the mind,' said one of the great Yogis of ancient times.

With a still mind, you can concentrate on what it is you want to achieve. It helps you to be single-minded, and single-mindedness is the best way to achieve your particular goals. With a still mind, you will have inner calm and peace instead of inner turmoil and inner hostilities.

The body's healing process works better when you are in a

positive state of mind, and yoga helps you get into a positive state of mind. If your mind is at peace, your body can be used to the best of its ability.

The idea of yoga is to still the mind, and be single-minded. It is important to grasp this, before doing the exercises, or asanas. 'Asana' literally means 'holding a position'. The asanas are postures in which you can hold your body while at the same time breathing correctly, quieting the mind, and being centre-pointed.

Meditation

One way to achieve a calm, still mind is meditation. You clear your mind of daily trivia and concentrate on just one thing. This one thing could be the breath, it could be a 'mantra' or chant, it could be a flower, for example. Meditation practised every day will help you feel calm and refreshed.

Transcendental Meditation

There have been some successes reported by people with MS using Transcendental Meditation. It has been known for people with quite severe disabilities to regain normal use of all their limbs and faculties by doing 20 minutes of TM a day.

For more information, look up TM in your local telephone directory.

Yoga Exercises for MS

People who think of yoga simply as a physical therapy will want to get on to the exercises, and to know how these can help them. But the exercises (or asanas) should not be thought of on their own. The correct yoga breathing, and the right mental approach, are as important as the exercises for your body. Howard Kent calls this the three Bs – brain, breath, and body. He says:

By the correct use of breathing and mental relaxation I have seen people move legs, with control, which have not moved in years; I have seen people get up from the floor unaided for the first time in years. Once the inhibitions are removed, the body's real powers can reveal themselves.

Any book on yoga will show you that there is a vast range of yoga exercises, or asanas. None of them is harmful to people with MS. To what extent these can be practised depends on the individual and the degree of disability.

When people with MS first start yoga, they often find it difficult to do a particular movement or hold a position. With practice, however, many people with MS find that they can make dramatic progress, and discover quite quickly that they can do some exercises they never thought possible.

If you have never done yoga before, it is hard to learn how to do it from a book. It is far better to go to a class. If you go to an ordinary yoga class, tell the teacher you have MS. You may find you cannot do some of the balance exercises at first (such as standing on one leg with your hands in a prayer position). But you may well be able to do them with a bit of practice.

There are classes specifically for people with MS run by the Yoga for Health Foundation. They have groups all over the country. Write to them at their headquarters to find out if there is a group in your area. They also run residential yoga holidays (weekends, weeks, or longer) at their HQ in the country, which is a beautiful old country house. The address is:

Yoga for Health Foundation
Ickwell Bury
Nr Biggleswade
Bedfordshire SG18 9EF
Tel: 01767 627271

Exercises to Do at Home

Once you have learned some basic exercises in a class, you can do them at home on your own. Ideally, to get the best out of it, you should practise yoga every day for at least 15 minutes.

Remember that yoga asanas tone up the neuro-muscular system of the body and keep it in full working order; they develop and control the respiratory system, increasing oxygen flow and vitality. The internal organs work better; the spine is kept strong and supple; you enjoy a sense of real well-being.

16

Mental Attitude

Any disability in your body will almost inevitably have some disabling effect on your mind. Your whole identity as a person is bound up with how you feel about yourself. And when your body does not do the things it used to do, you are likely to feel worse about yourself.

The trauma of being told you have MS is made worse by the fact that people think that multiple sclerosis must mean an inevitable downward slide into paralysis and a wheelchair.

That scenario is not necessarily true. Everything in this book is based on the real possibility of being able to halt that downward slide of MS if you start a self-help programme as soon as possible.

If you are early on in the disease, and not yet noticeably disabled, it is most important that you put in your mind's eye a mental picture of yourself in the future as someone who is healthy, active, and independent. Do not give house room in your mind to a future picture of yourself as someone ill, crippled, and with a life that has fallen apart.

The mental pictures you conjure up in your mind are incredibly powerful, without you realizing it. They have a way of being self-fulfilling. Concentrate your mind all the time on being healthy, strong, and active. Will yourself to stay well.

Knowing there are self-help therapies that work, and knowing there are countless numbers of people with MS who have *improved*, rather than got worse, as a result of following particular therapies, should make you feel more positive about things. You can hope for the best rather than for the worst.

BODY IMAGE

Unlike people born with a handicap, everyone with MS can easily remember all the things they could do before they had the disease. Everyone with MS was at one time fit and healthy, able to run around, play sports, sprint to catch a bus, leap up and down stairs, dance, and do all those other things you take for granted until you find you can't do them any longer.

When things like that become impossible, your body image changes, sometimes dramatically. People with MS come to see themselves as no longer useful or attractive to others. They must also learn to live with what is still the stigma of MS. A poor self-image can cause them to fear rejection by their partner, or prospective partners. By thinking this, it can happen.

Despite your symptoms and disabilities, it is important to try and keep hold of a positive body image. MS is no excuse for not taking care of your appearance, even if money is short. Many women I know with MS are beautiful and elegant, even though they may be in a wheelchair or walking with the aid of sticks.

REACTIONS TO MS

The counsellor at the MS Research Unit, Julia Segal, compiled a paper called *Reactions to MS* (available from ARMS), gleaned from the experience of ARMS in counselling hundreds of people with MS.

Julia Segal concludes 'There is MS . . . and there is the *reaction to MS*. The reaction to MS can be more destructive than the MS itself.' But the reaction to the MS can be affected by support from other people and counselling. People faced with the diagnosis of MS can react in different ways – their strategies for dealing with this disaster can vary.

Denial

One common strategy is denial – if you pretend you haven't got MS, it will go away. The thought processes of someone who chooses to deny they have MS will go something like this:

I don't tell people . . . they couldn't cope with it . . . I couldn't
cope with their pity . . . I'm afraid if I rest I will never get
up again . . . people will think I'm lazy . . . I make excuses
rather than tell people it's MS . . .

A common reason given for the denial approach is that people with
MS fear they will lose their job if their employer finds out they have
MS. This might be a well-founded fear in some cases, although
you might be surprised how helpful your employer is.

Another reason why people prefer to sweep their MS under the
carpet is because there is still, unfortunately, a fair amount of
stigma attached to MS. Once you declare you have MS, your status
as a person in society seems to go down. People do behave towards
disabled people differently. Everyone has seen the 'Does he take
sugar?' kind of behaviour, where if you're sitting in a wheelchair
people assume you can't speak for yourself.

Many people with MS lead a sort of double life. They tell some
people, but not others. They are likely to confide everything to
other people with MS, and turn to them for support and advice.
Yet they may say nothing about their MS to the world at large, to
their family members, and employers.

With this strategy, there is always the risk of being found out.
And of course, it only works if your disabilities don't give you away
to the people you want to keep it from.

Few people like others to feel sorry for them. But once you
declare to the world that you have MS, people are likely to respond
to you with 'Oh, poor you!' They are also quite likely to ring up
other friends and commiserate about your misfortune: 'Isn't it
terrible about poor John!' So instead of just being John, or Jane,
you are 'poor John' in the eyes of others.

Pretending that you haven't got MS is a hard act to keep up,
because you're always under the strain of hiding something from
other people. But even so, there might be some good practical
reasons to keep up the pretence until you absolutely have to reveal
the truth. It's a common strategy for the period following
diagnosis, a sort of holding strategy, until you decide what you're
going to do.

Julia Segal argues that there is a price to pay if you continue
to pretend that you haven't got MS. Friends will melt away,
because it's clear you didn't trust them; you will find yourself more
and more socially isolated, as your attitude may be pushing people

away from you. You are denying other people the choice of whether they want to be with you or not. It is very stressful always putting on a pretence. Also, you might be foolishly denying yourself help and support – both practical and emotional – that you really need.

MS as a Whole Identity

The other extreme to denying you have MS is letting MS take you over completely so it dominates your life. There are some people for whom multiple sclerosis becomes their whole identity. They have MS, but MS also has them.

After diagnosis, such people succumb to MS completely. They may give up work; they may go on disability pension; they may apply for a disabled sticker; they join some MS club; they meet other people less and less. They shift their whole life to a sub-culture of disabled people. MS becomes their hobby. They have no others.

Needing to meet and talk to other people with MS may be a very important stage that newly-diagnosed people have to go through. But making MS your whole life can create problems with families and friends.

I vividly remember the story of a man with MS who lived, breathed, slept MS. It was all he ever thought about or talked about. One day his wife screamed at him, 'If I ever hear the words MS again in this house I shall go stark staring mad!' This was a sufficient jolt for him to put MS into the context of his whole life, and lead a more balanced existence.

MS has become part of your life. But it is not your whole life. Dominate it before it dominates you.

MS as an Excuse

Another strategy which I have noticed in quite a few people with MS is using MS as an excuse for opting out of life as it should be lived. For example, a friend asks you to go out for a day in the country. You say, 'Sorry, I can't, I've got MS.' You really want to go, but you fear that your MS symptoms will make the day problematic. MS *does* get in the way. The symptoms are real. But some of the fears about the symptoms make them severe only in your head. By using MS as an excuse, you are denying yourself many opportunities to have a nice, or interesting, or pleasurable, time.

Depression

Depression is a much more common reaction to a diagnosis of MS than euphoria, which has been said to go with having MS.

Depression is most likely to happen soon after diagnosis, when the full implications of the disease hit you. If you have seen people in advanced stages of the disease, or you have read medical textbooks about MS, you may fear the worst is going to happen to you and so become awash with gloom and despair.

Depression is paticularly bad for someone with MS because it weakens an already weakened immune system. Your state of mind has a direct effect on your state of health.

It is not easy to counteract depression, but one Australian woman I know succeeds in keeping depression at bay with a simple 5-point plan:

1. Get plenty of sleep. Never get over-tired. (Notice how much more depressed and irritable you feel when you are tired.)
2. Eat often and plenty. Never allow yourself to get weak with hunger.
3. Exercise at least once a day. Exercise boosts your circulation, gets oxygen into your brain, and stokes up the body chemistry so that endorphins – the well-being hormones – are released.
4. Always have something to look forward to. Having MS can be like living in a dark tunnel. Always have treats in store to bring some sunshine into your life.
5. Be sociable. Take an interest in other people. This takes your mind off you and your troubles. Having MS is not a sentence to social isolation.

Add to that list:

6. Think positively.
7. Take care to look good. You can only feel good about yourself if you feel you look good.
8. Stick to as ordered a routine as you can and keep on top of things. That way you know where you are.
9. Keep your mind active and interested.

10. Do something that gives you a sense of achievement, for example a creative hobby, or helping other people in the community. Being proud of what you do is a great booster to the spirits.
11. Live in the present and get the most out of each experience as it is actually happening. Do not dwell on the past or be fearful about the future.

Some people have actually felt that getting MS is a blessing in disguise. Sometimes such people are religious. For them, having MS has made them truly appreciate some things in life which they used to take for granted. These are the people who derive new-found joy from the scent of a flower or the beauty of a tree. They strip from their lives all the nonsense that clutters up most people's daily existence, and instead just concentrate on the truly important things.

Life is lived slowly but richly. People who are able to rush because they can move fast miss the beauty of the rose petals.

Illness as an Opportunity to Change Your Life

One of the most positive approaches towards illness comes from the American surgeon Bernie Siegel in his two excellent books *Love, Medicine and Miracles* and *Peace, Love and Healing* (both published by Rider). I urge you to read them both.

In Bernie Siegel's view, 'exceptional patients' are those who do not see their illness as a disaster, but rather an opportunity to reassess their lives, change direction if necessary, but above all to live life to the full.

Somebody once said that the point of life is death. You literally need a deadline to make life very precious. Faced suddenly by your own mortality does give you a jolt to sort out your values and decide what your life should be all about.

Life is for living. Having MS does help you decide whether you'll opt to make the most of it, or squander it.

Self-Esteem

Self-esteem is your most vital asset. MS can dent it more visibly than a limp in your walk.

The most off-putting thing to other people is not that you walk with a limp or drag your left foot, but that you look downcast, grim-faced, embittered, or ready to bite anyone's head off if they speak to you.

Of course, when you have MS, it is easy to feel damaged, a psychological as well as a physical cripple, a second-rate person. Yet, this negative attitude is probably the most disabling thing of all. It is vital to fight it off.

Self-esteem is so important because people always think of you the same way you think of yourself. If you lack self-respect, you will not win respect from other people. If you are filled with self-loathing, you can be sure of a few enemies. If you have no love for yourself, no one else will be able to love you either. This is one of the hardest facts of life – but true.

Negative Thoughts and Feelings

Negative thoughts and feelings are known to undermine the health, lower the body's resistance to infection, and delay the healing process.

A negative personality is one who is lacking in self-confidence and full of self-doubt. They say 'no' rather than 'yes'. They say 'I can't' rather than 'I can'. They always imagine the most pessimistic outcome of any event. They are afraid of everything. They have no faith in their own powers, so they always go to other people for help. They tend to fail because they have an attitude which says 'it can't work'. They tend to see the worst in everything and everybody. They are very good at complaining, and forecasting doom and gloom.

Many people will hate to admit that they recognize themselves, or some of themselves some of the time, in this portrait. A negative personality, who only has negative thoughts and feelings, cannot be happy. Not only will he be unhappy, he will also be unwell, as this kind of negative programming is incompatible with good health.

You know from your own experience how the emotions can affect your body. Winning something makes you feel on top of the world, whereas bad news makes you feel ill, with perhaps symptoms of sickness, palpitations, a dry mouth, weakness, and so on.

The negative emotions all have a bad effect on your health.

Rage, fear, grief, sorrow, fright, jealousy, despondency, or pessimism make you feel bad physically. Of these, fear is supposed to be the most noxious.

On the other hand, the positive emotions of love, joy, and compassion make you feel good physically.

When you're told you have MS it is almost impossible to avoid feeling a wide range of negative emotions. Fear, grief, anger, rage, terror, shock, bewilderment, are all common feelings, particularly at the beginning.

A sense of loss is very common after you have been told you have MS. It is as if part of you has died, and you naturally mourn and grieve for it. The period of bereavement for your old self will take time. But the fear may linger on.

If negative feelings and emotions are getting the better of you, seek help. Bottling things up will only make things worse. There are various ways available which will help shift your emphasis away from the negative and towards the positive. These include yoga, meditation, visualization, psychotherapy, and counselling.

Visualization

Visualization techniques have become well known through the work of the Simontons and other cancer doctors in the USA, who have been using them to good effect in cancer treatment. Cancer patients were originally told to imagine things like white knights (white blood cells) killing the evil cancer cells, though recently less aggressive images have proved more acceptable.

It would be possible to use similar techniques in multiple sclerosis. The mind is very powerful, and the mental images you conjure up in your head can be translated into real life.

The best position for visualization is sitting erect (if possible) and breathing deeply. How you imagine your MS being overcome is up to you. Perhaps instead of conjuring up the image of the body's troops driving out the enemy, you may prefer to imagine pictures of yourself. In your mind's eye, always picture yourself happy, healthy, and active. You could imagine yourself swimming, or running along a beautiful beach, climbing mountains, or whatever.

This technique of intensely imagining yourself doing something active has worked in some cancer cases. It is also a technique used more and more to achieve success in competitive sport – players go through the mental process of, say, scoring a goal. Once you've rehearsed something carefully in your mind, it's much more likely to happen in real life. Don't allow house room in your head of pictures of yourself worse than you are now.

Fears

Counsellor Julia Segal has found that everyone with MS has a different worst fear about MS, and that talking your fears over with a trained counsellor is the best way of dealing with it. In her paper *Reactions to MS*, she lists some of the things people are most afraid of:

• Being in a wheelchair.
• Nobody finding you attractive any more.
• Being totally paralysed.
• Being cut off from everyone.
• Going blind and being alone in the dark.
• Waking up one morning unable to move.

With counselling, it is possible to talk these fears through and realize that there is a less stark side to each of these scenarios. Firstly, it hasn't happened yet and might never happen. Secondly, the fears themselves are probably unrealistic. For example, men do still flirt with women in wheelchairs if they have attractive personalities and take a pride in their appearance.

COUNSELLING

Counselling really can help. People can be helped to feel and behave better. Anxieties are brought out into the open, and are possible to solve with the help of a trained counsellor. It is very important that someone with MS feels they have someone to turn to.

Counselling someone with MS can help in the following ways:

• Work with a counsellor can re-establish the ability to enjoy life. The counsellor can help deal with the anger which is preventing recognition of real pleasures and remaining abilities.

- Counselling can uncover hidden love. Resentment and anger arising out of the MS can cover up and bury real love and affection. Counselling can help people to find, recognize, and express their love again.
- Counselling can sometimes help lift depression and stop the person with MS from seeming to punish the family, and so making them feel guilty.

The Multiple Sclerosis Society runs three telephone counselling services (see page 193).

The MS Society also has an MS Helpline which provides information and support. They have a large database of information and can help with all aspects of MS, Social Security benefits, help from social services, aids and equipments, respite centres, holidays, etc.

MS Helpline: 0171-371 8000

MEDITATION

Meditation is a proven way of learning to control the way stress affects us. Meditation helps to focus on the present moment and not dwell on the past or worry about the future. Anxiety and negative thoughts are hostile to the immune system, and meditation can help counteract these. It is thought that regular practice – 20 minutes a day – particularly in the relapsing/remitting form of MS, not only reduces the number of relapses but also their severity. It also calms the mind, brings mental clarity, improves concentration, and helps you become a more positive person.

Transcendental Meditation centres are listed in telephone directories. Steve Brisk, who has MS and says his life has changed through relaxation and meditation, runs courses and has made two cassettes: *Gentle on Your Mind: Deep Relaxation*, and *How to Meditate, Beat Stress and Improve Your Health*. Both are sold through the MS Society, and available from its headquarters at £6.95 each. Cheques should be made payable to MSS (Trading) Ltd.

For his courses, contact Steve directly:

Steve Brisk
33 Beverley Gardens, Woodmancote, Cheltenham GL52 4QD.
Tel: 01243 674006

The Metaphysics of Illness

Some psychologists think that each physical illness has a mental cause; each physical illness has a particular attitude or set of attitudes which go to make up the personality of the person who has that illness. Nowadays, 'the cancer personality' is a phrase which people understand.

In the United States, the metaphysics of illness has quite a following. One of the handbooks of this approach is *Heal Your Body* by Louise L. Hay. For each physical condition, she lists a probable metaphysical cause, and the new thought pattern which will overcome the problem.

Problem	Probable Cause	New Thought Pattern
Multiple Sclerosis	Mental hardness, hard-heartedness, iron will, inflexibility.	I no longer try to control, I flow along with the joy of life.

* Published by Louise L. Hay, 11906 Goshen Avenue, Los Angeles, CA 90049

Louise Hay has since written *You Can Heal Your Life* (published by Hay House, USA) in which she describes how changing your thought patterns can, literally, heal you.

A similar metaphysical approach is taken by the American authors of *Health for the Whole Person* published by Westview Press (editors Hastings, Fadiman and Gordon).

A person with MS is described as having the following attitude:

'This person feels forced to undertake some kind of physical activity and does not want to. He has to work without help, has to support himself and usually others. He does not want to, and wishes help or support.

You might feel that neither of these descriptions of an 'MS attitude' accurately describes yourself. Even so, you might feel that examining your thought processes and attitudes to see whether they need changing is a worthwhile thing to do.

17

Hints on Daily Living

MS symptoms can come and go, even within one day. Sometimes it seems there is neither rhyme nor reason why you should feel worse today than you did yesterday. However, there are some things which can bring on MS symptoms, and so should be avoided as much as possible. These include humid heat, hot baths, over-exertion, stressful events, over-tiredness, and hunger.

This chapter also gives hints on how to deal with some of the unwanted symptoms of MS which affect daily life, such as fatigue, constipation, and incontinence. It also says why habits such as drinking and smoking are so bad for you when you have MS.

When you do have MS, you should try and do everything to maintain the best health possible. The diet and exercise advice already given would help that. But nutrition and exercise alone are not enough.

HOMOEOSTASIS

One of the oldest concepts of good health, going back to Hippocrates, is homoeostasis. Nowadays we might call this balance, or harmony. What quickly becomes apparent once you have MS is that the area in which you can maintain homoeostasis shrinks.

Before you had MS, you could probably tolerate extremes of temperature without too much complaint; you could probably tolerate a humid summer; you could probably go Christmas

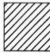 Area of
normal
homoeostasis

Figure 15: Homoeostasis

shopping without flaking out; you could probably work long hours when you needed to without feeling like a radio with run-down batteries.

But once you have MS, you look at other people and marvel at what they can do. They have the health and energy to do things which seem impossible to you now.

The area within which healthy people still feel healthy and energetic is considerably greater than for most people with MS. In other words, what will maintain homoeostasis in a healthy person is not what will maintain homoeostasis in someone with MS.

The possibilities do become limited. The kind of work you do, your family commitments, how you get around, where you live, where you go on holiday, and what type of holiday you have are all quite seriously affected by having MS.

You have to find out for yourself what conditions will maintain your homoeostasis, and what circumstances go dangerously outside it. These will differ from person to person.

For example, I know that for me the ideal temperature to maintain my own homoeostasis is around 65°F, with no humidity. Once it goes above 75°F, with any humidity, I feel like the proverbial wet dishcloth and cannot function properly.

I have also had to impose similar limits regarding how far I can drive in one go; how many hours I can work; how late I can stay up, etc. My own limited sphere of homoeostasis corresponds roughly with the small box in Figure 15. The old me, pre-MS, could operate very well within the bigger box.

I do find that I can remain stable as long as I stay within this small box. The trouble starts when I try and go beyond it.

FATIGUE

Fatigue is one of the most insidious symptoms of MS, and one which has devastating effects in almost every area of life. It may make it impossible for you to carry on working full time; it makes it more difficult to bring up a family.

Fatigue in MS is not like normal fatigue, from which you can recuperate quite easily with a good rest. It is chronic fatigue, where everything seems to be an effort. Even simple things, like hanging out the washing, become daunting tasks.

Fatigue in MS is not just tired muscles. It is the effect of the disease on the nerves which go to the muscles; and also the effect of the disease on the sensory nerves. The sensory nerves affect touch, sight, taste, smell and hearing. So when you get fatigued, you can sometimes experience blurring of vision or slurring of speech.

What happens when you get fatigued can differ from person to person. Fatigue often worsens existing symptoms, or can bring on symptoms which only happen when you are fatigued. Also, old symptoms can come back, with the nasty habit of reminding you of your last attack. Severe fatigue can also bring on episodes of vertigo, where the ceiling spins. You can also feel ill, as if you have flu.

There are certain things which can bring on fatigue, as well as other MS symptoms. When you know what these things are, fatigue is easier to avoid.

What brings on fatigue can differ from person to person. However, some of the most common things are: a hot day, humid weather, a hot bath, over-exertion, over-tiredness, a heavy meal, smoking, and stress. Fatigue can also be one of the major symptoms of a food allergy.

Why Do You Get Fatigued?

Any movement of any muscle requires energy. Energy starts from glucose, and to convert glucose into energy the muscle needs oxygen.

Oxygen is brought to the muscle by the blood circulating through it. If there is not enough oxygen because of poor circulation, substances like lactic acid accumulate, and prevent the muscles from working. The oxygen supply to the muscles is increased when the blood flow is improved by exercise.

Of course, the whole process of energy production and muscle contraction is a highly complex one. However, it is important to understand the essential link between blood-flow, oxygen, and the working of the muscles.

Fatigue happens when the blood flow, hence the oxygen flow to the muscles, is inadequate.

Exercise to Combat Fatigue

If you are physically fit, you have a better chance of withstanding fatigue. To keep fit, you must keep the muscles exercised. You should never exercise to the point of exhaustion, and should stop before feeling tired or hot. However, if you do not do any exercise at all, you will get fatigued much more easily than if you do.

Exercise tones up the whole system (see chapter 14). After a session of gym, yoga, or swimming, for example, you should have more energy, not less.

Your body will give you early warning signals as to when it is time to stop and rest.

An excellent book on overcoming fatigue is *The Beat Fatigue Workbook* by leading naturopath Leon Chaitow, published by Thorsons. It goes into great detail as to all the things one can do to counteract fatigue, many of them nutritional.

HEAT AND HUMIDITY

A common experience with MS is to become very sensitive to heat, particularly humid heat. Hot, humid summers can be hell for someone with MS, who feels weak and drained all the time with no energy for anything.

It is important to keep cool. Air conditioning would be very nice if you could afford it. A fan in every room is a second best.

Dry heat seems to be tolerated by people with MS, and many enjoy being in not too hot sunshine, as long as there is no humidity. Where you choose to go for your holiday becomes an issue. It may be better to go on holiday off-season, when it is not too hot.

Be very careful with hot baths. They can bring on MS symptoms very rapidly, as well as leaving you very weak. These symptoms tend to go away once the effects of the hot bath have worn off, but are unpleasant nevertheless. They can be avoided by making sure that the bath water is comfortably warm, but not hot.

OVER-EXERTION

One of the problems about having MS is that many people – particularly those who are young and energetic – want to prove that they can still do all the things they used to. So they over-compensate, and make themselves ill by over-exertion.

Young people with MS who have not told their employer, their workmates, or even their family, are more at risk of over-exertion. Driving a lorry from London to Scotland in one haul may be fine if you are a fit and healthy man, but it's simply asking for trouble if you have MS and are hiding it from everyone.

The ones who seem to suffer most from over-exertion are wives. Women stricken with MS have, in my view, the toughest time because in our so-called emancipated society they are often expected to do three full-time jobs: go out to work, run the household, and be a mother.

The 'energy cake' when you have MS is not enough to fulfil even one of these roles properly, let alone three.

I have received letters from wives which have made my blood boil. Even though the wife has MS, the husbands still expect them to cook, clean, look after the children, *and* go out to work to help earn a living.

Time and time again, women in that situation are called 'lazy' if they do not visibly do all the chores. A woman with MS may feel so weak after a day at work she is only fit to slump in the armchair. Not wanting to be labelled 'lazy' or 'selfish', many of these women force themselves to cook a meal, clean the house, do the laundry, the ironing, or whatever. The kind of chores which women are expected to do are particularly energy-consuming. The easiest place to suffer from over-exertion is in the home. Fatigue is the likely result.

Many women suffer this kind of unfair treatment from their families because they may *look* perfectly OK. The 'invisible' symptoms of MS, such as fatigue, are not obvious to other people in the same way that a limp, or a hacking cough, is.

Continual over-exertion such as this can only lead to trouble; worsening symptoms are almost inevitable as there is no let-up in the constant strain.

The workload simply has to be shared with other people, somehow, or lessened, or both. This kind of situation may need relationship counselling, and/or help from the social services, if you can get it.

MS will almost certainly mean altering the traditional roles in your household, and this will take time to adjust.

WORK

Over-exertion is often tied up with the work you do. Many people find that their job is simply not compatible with having MS. For example, a surveyor could not continue to climb up on roofs or balance along parapet walls. Two journalists I know could not carry on rushing about everywhere and meeting tight deadlines; a pilot I knew had to forget about flying planes. The list is endless.

Once you have MS, your 'energy cake' is much smaller, and you have to choose how you are going to share it out. It probably means setting your sights lower. It will probably mean watching your contemporaries being promoted over your head, when you can see that – if things had turned out differently – it could have been you being promoted.

One of the most painful things about MS is that it does strike at young people in their prime. This is just the age when people are aiming to make it in their chosen career or walk of life. It hurts to see success, and probably fortune too, being snatched from your grasp. This is particularly so at a period when someone's whole identity – male or female – is so bound up with the work they do.

Even if you succeed in not getting worse, even if you successfully stabilize the disease, you will probably still have to sacrifice some work. If your present job is strenuous and stressful, you will have to weigh up whether the price you will have to pay in fatigue is worth it. If you carry on working full-time in a demanding job, you may be too tired to do anything else when you come home. The idea is probably to find some suitable part-time work, if possible, or change to a less demanding job which is full-time, even if it means stepping down a few rungs in the career ladder.

You do not have to give up work altogether because you have MS. It is likely to be pretty damaging to your self-esteem and self-confidence – as well as to your pocket – if you do. Try and find the right balance between work and the rest of your life.

OVER-TIREDNESS

If you feel tired (not the same as fatigue), then rest. If you don't rest, it may turn into fatigue all too easily.

A rest some time during the day is highly desirable. If you can manage twice a day, so much the better. It will feel like recharging your batteries. You don't have to go to sleep. Just lie down and relax completely. You could read a book, or meditate. You will feel more relaxed if you put your feet up.

SLEEP

If you are going short of sleep, you are bound to feel fatigued. Try to go to bed early.

Tell yourself you will be in bed by a particular time every night, with perhaps one late night a week. This means being firm with other people. If you are invited out anywhere, politely insist on leaving when you feel it is time for you to go. It will doubtless happen that your host or hostess will make you feel guilty about leaving so 'early', but guilt is better than fatigue.

If you can manage it, get some sleep during the day. An hour or so after lunch is usually the best time. Some symptoms of MS go away almost miraculously after a good sleep.

EATING

A woman I know with MS gave me some invaluable advice which works like magic in some instances of fatigue – eat and drink plenty and often.

Being 'weak with hunger' has a particular relevance to MS people. The symptoms of that unnatural fatigue (what some people call 'feeling MSy') creep over you when you begin to feel hungry, and get worse as you get hungrier. If you go without breakfast, you could be feeling deathly by mid-morning.

Of all the things that bring on fatigue, this is the easiest to overcome. At home, you have instant access to the fridge or larder (stick to nutritious snacks, not junk food). Problems arise when you go out. Some people serve dinner late and your legs could be like jelly by the time the soup is served. Far better to eat a little something before you leave the house. If you're going on a journey, take emergency rations with you.

There's no need to stuff yourself, or get fat; simply plug the hole in your stomach before you get really hungry and weak. But don't make the mistake of eating sugary foods, as your blood sugar level will rise sharply, then dip.

Blood Sugar Levels

In fact a common cause of fatigue is hypoglycaemia – low blood sugar level. Unless you are aware of hypoglycaemia, it would be easy just to say 'I feel fatigued' without realizing the cause – or the solution. The way to avoid hypoglycaemia is to eat complex carbohydrates (e.g. wholemeal pasta) little and often. This gives a slow release of glucose into the bloodstream. The worst thing is to eat sugary foods, for the reason given above.

How to Eat Properly

Eating properly may sound trivial, but it is in fact vitally important to good health.

Here are some general guidelines:

1. Chew all your food slowly and thoroughly

Chewing tears your food apart with your teeth, and the food mixes with saliva in your mouth, which is the first stage in the digestive process. It is not good to swallow lots of unchewed food, as it gives the digestive substances a hard time. The more thoroughly you chew, the greater the amount of nutrients your body will absorb.

Semi-digested food particles passing through the gut wall may be involved in allergic reactions and other symptoms of ill-health.

2. Ideally, do not drink with meals

Too much fluid with food interferes with the digestive substances. Ideally, do not drink any fluids from at least half an hour before any meal, nor until half an hour after that meal.

3. Drink at least five glasses of water a day

When you are thirsty, drink water in preference to anything else. Go for pure bottled still spring water or filtered tap water. Still water is better than the artificially carbonated waters. Do not drink ice-cold water.

4. Rotate Your Foods

Food rotation means eating a particular food only once in every four days. This applies particularly to the grains containing gluten, which are wheat, barley, oats, and rye.

A seasonal diet, of foods eaten only in season, would be ideal to keep our bodies attuned and allow the digestive enzymes recovery time. But of course this is virtually impossible today.

A break of four days between foods gives the liver time to process any toxin from a food group, and for the enzymes to recuperate fully.

By rotating foods, you are assured of fully digesting the food you take in, leading to less toxic waste.

5. Attempt to Eat in a Biochemical Balance

Aim for a biochemical balance between acid and alkaline foods, and between cooked and raw foods. You might need a macrobiotic cook book to help you discover which foods are acid and which are alkaline. If you choose foods from opposite polarities, it helps the body stay balanced.

6. Food Combining for Health

Ideally, do not eat protein with starches, and do not eat fruit with protein meals. There are several books about food combining which explain the health benefits of it.

Weight

In fact, despite the advice about eating, it is sensible to lose weight if you are overweight. This is because if you are carrying around surplus weight you will get fatigued more quickly. A nutritious, low animal fat diet, even one high in complex carbohydrates, will not make you put on weight.

Food Allergies

Fatigue is one of the classic symptoms of food allergies. Ironically, the time you are most likely to get symptoms from an allergic food is *not* just after eating the offending food, but when you have not eaten the offending food for a while. This is called a 'masked allergy'. Some people find that their fatigue disappears once they have identified and excluded the foods to which they are allergic. (See chapter 9.)

SMOKING

Smoking has very bad effects on MS. It can cause worsening of MS symptoms. One of the frequent effects of smoking is to lower skin temperature. This can aggravate MS, where people tend to suffer from a feeling of cold in the hands and feet anyway. Also, eye problems in MS can sometimes be associated with smoking.

Everyone knows that smoking can cause lung cancer, bronchitis and emphysema, and cardiovascular disorders.

The toxic substances from a single cigarette, such as cadmium, lower the blood level of vitamin C and destroy about 25 mg of the vitamin.

Smoking can only do you harm. It is one of the greatest health hazards, and the most preventable cause of premature death.

Smoking also interferes with the beneficial effects of a diet high in essential fatty acids.

So, *don't smoke.*

DRINKING ALCOHOL

Alcohol can worsen MS symptoms, which can sometimes make you look a bit like a drunk anyway. Alcohol can make co-ordination worse, and may affect standing, walking, finger movements, eye movements and speech. Far from being a stimulant, alcohol acts as a depressant. It could well make you feel low rather than high.

In some diets for MS, for example the Swank Diet, alcohol is allowed in *small quantities.* If you find that a glass of good wine or sherry does not make you feel ill, there's no harm in drinking them occasionally.

However, a lot of alcohol can do you harm. In inhibits the conversion process of the essential fatty acids, and nothing should get in the way of this vital process.

Alcohol causes the amount of saturated fat in the blood to increase. It increases the need for vitamin B1, pantothenic acid, and choline.

Be careful in case you have an allergy to some of the ingredients in alcoholic drinks. Sugar is added to many alcoholic drinks. Yeast is added to some.

Alcohol is probably the most difficult thing to refuse socially. Everyone expects everyone else to drink, and a glass of something is always being shoved in your hand at parties. However, if drink does make you feel ill, you must resist this kind of pressure. Insist on mineral water, or pure unsweetened fruit juices.

CONSTIPATION

Constipation is a common complaint in MS. It is something that it is important to remedy, because continued constipation has many bad effects; there is a build-up of toxins in the system; the full bowel presses on the bladder and makes you more likely to be incontinent; you feel horribly bunged-up.

Fibre

The ARMS EFA diet (chapter 6) is high in fibre, or roughage. High fibre foods include: onions, parsnips, celery, peas, beans, stringy vegetables – all raw or lightly cooked; whole grains, wholemeal bread; bran; oatmeal; nuts; fresh and dried fruits.

The ARMS diet also recommends additional bran, to be sprinkled on breakfast cereals, fruit purées, low-fat yogurts, etc.

Refined foods are low in fibre and can only make constipation worse, not better.

Psyllium seed husks

Another excellent fibre is psyllium seed husks. These are a valuable source of non-digestible plant fibre. As much as one tablespoon can be taken with each meal, until bowel regulation occurs. Then the amount can be reduced to one or two teaspoons, three times a day, every fourth day (so as to rotate this fibre with other fibre foods on a 4-day rotation basis). Psyllium seed husks are available from chemists.

When you are eating a high fibre diet, it is most important to drink a lot of water. The fibre needs the water to pass easily along the bowel.

In fact, water is probably the most important anti-constipation agent there is. The first thing to do if you are not regular, is to drink as much water as possible. Make a habit of drinking one glassful when you get up.

Evening Primrose Oil

Many people have found that their constipation has been relieved after taking evening primrose oil capsules. The frequent use of oils like sunflower seed oil in salad dressing and cooking will help too.

Linusit Gold

Linusit Gold is a brand of linseeds, easily found in health food shops. You can sprinkle it liberally on breakfast cereals, yogurt, salads and so on. It is excellent at helping to relieve constipation, and has the added bonus of being rich in alpha-linolenic acid.

Dried Fruit

Another tip is to chew whole fruit and dried fruit such as figs and take linseeds and/or stewed prunes before each meal.

Acidophilus

New research into intestinal flora ('probiotics') has found that bowel regularity has more to do with your intestinal flora, than with the amount of fibre you eat. Many people swear by taking acidophilus, a friendly bacteria found in the gut. This bacteria would be decimated if you were taking antibiotics.

Vitamin C

A good intake of vitamin C helps keep the stools soft – as much as 2-4 grams, three times a day. The use of vitamin C as a bowel softener has considerable value beyond the retention of fluid in the colon. It also serves as a detoxifying substance for toxins formed by bacteria in the colon.

If you are sagging in your posture, and sluggish generally, you are more likely to be constipated. Toning up the whole system by exercise will get you going in more ways than one.

Do not take laxatives. This makes the bowel lazy. It also means that your body loses much-needed vitamins and minerals. Continued use of laxatives can make you feel very unwell.

Finally, allow enough unhurried time on the toilet.

To sum up, combat constipation with:

- A high fibre diet including added bran.
- Lots of water. Start the day with a glass of water.
- Oils such as evening primrose oil or sunflower seed oil.
- Chew lots of whole fruit and dried fruits like figs.
- Take linseeds and/or stewed prunes before each meal.
- Take Linusit Gold on cereals etc.
- Take acidophilus capsules once a day.
- Unhurried time on the toilet.

BLADDER PROBLEMS

Of all the symptoms of MS, incontinence is probably the one people feel most miserable about.

When there is damage to the nerve pathways in the lower part of the spine, control of the bladder can be weakened. You may feel an urgent need to go to the toilet frequently, even though there is not much urine in the bladder.

Alternatively, some people suffer from bladder retention, when they cannot pass water, no matter how hard they try or how much they feel they want to go. In more advanced cases of MS, double incontinence (faecal incontinence) can sometimes happen too.

These are particularly distressing symptoms because they are surrounded in our society by feelings of embarrassment and shame. Some people I know with MS find the possibility of wetting themselves in public, not being able to find a toilet in time, or emitting an unpleasant odour, a worse handicap than, say, walking with a limp.

The present-day statistics are that 50-80 per cent of all MS patients experience bladder problems at some point.

However, there are many anecdotal cases of bladder symptoms clearing up when people have detected their food allergies and cut out the offending foods. Hyperbaric oxygen also helps bladder symptoms in some people.

You may find that if you stick to the self-help management programme in this book, you may not suffer from bladder problems at all. I have never suffered from any bladder problems myself (touch wood!)

Bladder symptoms often become worse than they need be because of simple neglect. A consultant urologist speaking at a recent symposium on MS said: 'I am sad to say that some of the greatest cases of neglect have been those with neuropathic disorders.' He was talking about MS specifically.

Patients may feel embarrassed to seek help about something still considered vaguely shameful. And doctors may not be referring patients to the right kind of help early enough.

Here again, we have a situation similar to that of secondary handicap. Contractures and deformities can happen to someone with MS, not as part of the disease process, but because they did not receive physiotherapy early enough. Likewise, many people with MS put up with agonizing symptoms, such as bladder urinary retention, when the right help could have saved them pain and misery. Bladder infections can be a secondary complication of bladder problems. But with the right help early enough, these can be avoided.

Secondary complications should never be allowed to happen. It is most important to deal with bladder problems like retention, and infection, before they can lead to anything worse.

There is now something called CISC – Clean Intermittent Self Catheterization – for patients who are not able to empty their bladders properly.

For the whole range of bladder symptoms, there is a range of drugs available on prescription from your doctor. So you should see your doctor, and ideally be asked to be referred to a consultant urologist at the nearest hospital where they have one. Some urology departments have incontinence counsellors.

With the help of drugs, possibly a catheter, possibly HBO, possibly special pants and pads, it is possible to manage the problem of incontinence in such a way as to lead a near-normal life.

There are many incontinence advisors at hospitals around the country. There is also research into incontinence going on at The National Hospital in London. Your GP may be able to refer you. Or get in touch with:

InconTact (National Action on Incontinence)
2 Doughty Street
London WC1N 2PH
Helpline: 0191-213 0050

Drinking

You might think if you cut down on your fluid intake, your need to rush to the toilet will be reduced. Not so. The trouble with drinking very little is that the urine becomes concentrated and smelly, which can create its own problems.

Ideally, you should drink at least five glasses of fluid a day, more (8–10) if possible. Drink more earlier in the day. Do not drink anything for a couple of hours before going to bed if you normally have to get up in the night to go to the toilet. That way, you are less likely to be up several times in the night. If you wear a catheter it is very important to drink a lot of fluid, otherwise it collects debris. A high fluid intake will prevent this.

Drinking a good amount is also an essential to avoid constipation. In fact, constipation itself can be a cause of stress incontinence, because the full bowel is pressing on the bladder (see section on constipation).

Both coffee and red wine can irritate the bladder lining and make you feel more of an urge to pass water than you would feel otherwise. Other alcoholic drinks could have the same effect too.

Going to the Toilet

It is common sense to organize your life so you are not far away from a toilet. Before setting out on a journey, or going somewhere you have never been before, it is a wise precaution to find out where the toilets are. You might prefer to avoid, for example, motorways which have no service stations on them.

Once in the toilet, make sure you empty your bladder completely. Stay there long enough to make sure there is nothing left. Women should lean forward to help empty the bladder thoroughly.

STRESS

Some doctors believe that trauma triggers MS in susceptible people. If you ask people with MS where they experienced their first symptom, many will describe a part of the body which suffered a trauma previous to the onset of MS.

Other people will say that there were very stressful events just before MS was diagnosed. Attacks, or relapses, of MS can often be caused by stress.

One definition of stress is not having the resources to meet the demands made on you. The more feeble your resources, the more stressful demands made on you will be. The more abundant your resources, the less stressful demands made on you will be.

Resources mean both practical resources, such as money and equipment, and inner resources, such as strength of will, and health. Obviously, if you are ill your inner resources will be depleted, and demands that would not feel like stress to a well person suddenly become stressful. So the more you can retain or regain your health and well being, the better you will be able to deal with stress.

Attitude is also very important. Remember that one person's stress is another person's challenge. Your personality, or how you respond to a particular situation, is perhaps more relevant than the stressor itself. For example, some people get a thrill from taking off in an aeroplane, while others find it stressful. Some people love working to deadlines, while others seize up at the thought of it.

If you can gain some insight into yourself and see that stress is making your symptoms worse, you could do one of two things. You could set about reducing these stresses from your life, or you could change your attitude to them (or both).

Many people with MS identify themselves as having very short fuses. Their ability to withstand even minor stress is diminished. If you can see that your reaction to stress is very pronounced, you might benefit from counselling or psychotherapy.

When you feel under stress, the hormones in your body become unbalanced. Cortisol, the hormone of hopelessness and helplessness, interferes with the metabolism of essential fatty acids. So you should try and relax, or reduce the circumstances which make you feel stressed.

HRT (Hormone Replacement Therapy)

No research has been done on HRT and women with MS. At an ARMS meeting in 1991, Dr John Studd, director of the menopause clinic at Dulwich Hospital in London, said that HRT seemed a good idea as it prevented osteoporosis and treated hot flushes. However, Dr Rosie Jones, working on MS research at Bristol Royal Infirmary, feels that she would be unhappy to recommend it. Some women with MS taking HRT have reported feeling more energetic with the bonus of young-looking skin, while some others have reported relapses which they felt were connected with the HRT. If you are a menopausal woman with MS, it would be worth discussing HRT seriously with a gynaecologist.

18

Relationships and Sex

Once you have MS, your relationships with everyone change – including with yourself. You are the one you have to go on living with, and you have to like your own company first before relationships will work with other people.

Having MS will affect your relationship with yourself, with your partner if you have one, and your ability to find a partner if you do not have one already.

Having MS will affect your relationships inside the family – with your children if you are a parent, or with your parents if you are the 'child' with MS. Brothers, sisters, and wider family will also be affected. So will friends, neighbours, work-mates, and employers if you have them. The ripples from having MS spread far and wide.

The ideal is that your MS is controlled and never gets bad. But the trouble with MS is that people with the disease live with the fear that deterioration is lurking round the next corner. So, even if you are only mildly disabled, the fact that you have MS is bound to affect all relationships – if you let it.

Perhaps the most damaging thing that MS can do is to make you feel bad about yourself. This is pernicious because the way you feel about yourself is crucial both to having rewarding relationships and a fulfilling sex life.

RELATIONSHIPS WITH A PARTNER

If you already have an intimate and loving relationship with your partner, there is no reason why MS should threaten the relationship; indeed, it could well bring you closer together.

On the other hand, a chronic and potentially disabling illness like MS can throw a severe strain on a relationship which lacks deep intimacy and communication. If the person with MS finds it difficult to talk freely and difficult to accept help, or is very demanding; or if the partner is unable to offer help, then a marriage could be in dire straits.

When either a husband or wife gets MS, it is difficult to carry on with family life as if nothing has happened. On the other hand, the person with MS does not want to be labelled as an invalid, and give up the role of wife, mother, husband, father, or breadwinner.

Even though your body image may have changed, you are still you. You are still able to give and receive love, to laugh, cry, share emotions, and be needed by your family, friends, and colleagues. You will feel more of a sense of worth if you keep reminding yourself that you are needed, loved and lovable.

If you go round being a misery and a grump, you will find it difficult to like yourself, and you can hardly expect others to like you either. A frown puts people off, but a smile attracts.

You can control your moods if you decide to. It is better to try and take a light-hearted approach to MS problems than a heavy-handed, gloomy one. Certainly, they are no joke, but the people I know with MS who can manage to make a joke out of their difficulties tend to get on much better in life than those who do not. They are the kind who might chuckle, 'Oh! There I go, peeing again!' when they are incontinent, rather than being shamefully embarrassed about it.

Relationship Problems

It is easy to turn MS into the scapegoat for all marital and sexual problems, when it is the basic relationship itself that is at fault.

Even so, MS is going to affect any relationship dramatically. Feelings that neither of you may have had to confront before are likely to hit you with a terrible impact: feelings of fear, frustration, rage, perhaps hostility and guilt.

Each couple must work out for themselves the issues of dependence and independence – to what extent the one with MS can make demands on the other, and to what extent the one without MS should give help to the other. Some sufferers will fall into the 'sick' role, and use it to manipulate their partners or other relatives, but this will only make them feel guilt and hostility.

These issues are very hard to deal with, but they must be confronted and talked through. It may be necessary to get help from a professional therapist or counsellor.

CHILDREN

Children can be very bewildered and shocked by a parent who gets MS. They may have had a mum who used to run round the park with them, or a dad who played football, but cannot any longer.

What and when you tell them depends on their age, but the key is to be honest. Try not to tell a four year-old more than he can understand. Instinctively, children are aware that something is wrong and that you are worried. You need to be aware of this and understand that their behaviour can sometimes be disturbed. They need comfort and reassurance.

Your children may have to alter their views about what mothers and fathers are supposed to be like, and this adjustment will take time.

Older children may appear outwardly calm or even indifferent when they are told you have MS, yet inwardly they could be acutely anxious about it. The way to deal with this is to talk to them, giving a little information at a time rather than one long talk. Treat them as adults, and let them play a responsible part in family life.

Children's Fears

Children can feel afraid if one of their parents has MS, but this fear may not be at the conscious level, says counsellor Julia Segal.

The deep-down terror is that their mum or dad is going to die because of MS; and that they themselves will get MS.

Children can also feel guilty that somehow they were responsible for their parents' MS, particularly if the first attack happened soon after their own birth.

Children do feel responsible for their parents; they may well feel that they are responsible for the life and death of their parents. They can easily have 'silly' thoughts, such as that if only they loved their mum and dad more, or properly, he or she would get better. They might think that if mum or dad is not getting better, it's because they don't love mum or dad enough. The conclusion from this thought process is that they are a very bad person because they cannot love mum or dad enough to make them better.

All these fears and anxieties can affect the child's behaviour. Either the child may pretend he doesn't care, or the child can be over-anxious to please.

The child who pretends not to care may be violent or aggressive. This might be interpreted as a way of saying 'It's not my fault'. It might also be a way of provoking the parent into anger, and so making him or her more alive.

The child who is always very anxious to please is always very helpful and afraid of doing the wrong thing. He is almost doing a role reversal. Instead of being the child who needs to be cared for, he tries to be the parent.

These deep-down fears and anxieties need to be brought out into the open if the child is not going to be disturbed. Ideally, this needs to be done with a professional therapist or counsellor.

WHO CARES FOR THE CARERS?

A new social problem has been highlighted recently in the UK by the Carers National Association – children caring for their disabled parents.

If the able-bodied parent has to go out to work, or has walked out on the family, it is not that unusual for some of the burden of care to fall on a child.

Even though in the UK there are social services, their first question is often to ask, 'Isn't there somebody in the family who can help?' Rather than send round a home help, or a social worker, to relieve the family, they leave it to the child or children in the family. Even children well under the age of majority are considered 'somebody in the family' as far as helping a disabled person is concerned.

It is not unusual to find children doing the shopping, helping with the cooking, helping with the housework, and taking their disabled parent to the toilet in the night – all this on top of going to school and perhaps doing homework.

In situations such as these, the child in question is often faced with a triple trauma: one parent has MS and is ill; the other parent has walked out because of this; the child cannot do what normal children do because he or she has to do household and nursing duties.

Children in situations such as this cannot go out to play with other children, because they feel they cannot leave the disabled parent alone – in case they need to go to the toilet, in case something happens, in case they need something.

This forces quite young children to be grown up before they have finished their childhood. It may make them into mature, helpful, altruistic adults. But it could also leave them resentful that they are sacrificing what they *really want* to do for something they really *don't want* to do.

As the years roll by, the child turns into a teenager, and then a young adult. At this point the disabled parent often feels a terrible burden on his own child – that he is getting in the way of that child leading a social life, going out and enjoying him or herself, even meeting someone and getting married.

None of these problems has easy solutions, and each individual solution will be different. Generally, the more help you can get from other people, the less likely it is that the children will have to bear an undue burden on their own.

THE PROBLEMS FOR PARENTS IF THEIR CHILD HAS MS

Of course, the situation can often be the other way around – the child (of whatever age) has MS, and the parent has to face that tragedy.

How can you help your parents accept your illness without any feelings of guilt on their part, or blame on your part?

If you think that there was something they did or did not do during your first fifteen or so years of life, you can easily feel that it's your parents' fault that you have MS. Maybe your mother fed you the wrong diet, maybe she weaned you too early, maybe one of your parents passed on some genetic predisposition. Thoughts such as these may very well enter your mind.

All these thoughts are likely to be going through the parent's head as well: 'If only I had done/not done this or that, this might never have happened.'

The blame/guilt feelings may very well affect the relationship between the MS sufferer and his or her parents; even if those actual emotions never come out into the open, they are still there, festering underneath.

If the person develops MS before he or she has found a partner and got married, it may fall on the parents to look after that child long after his or her childhood is over. All parents want the best for their child, and want to care for him as much as they can. The problems arise when the child is no longer a child but a young adult who wants independence from his parents, and who does not want to be mollycoddled.

Being looked after by your parents once you are grown up is very demoralizing for some people. They do not want to be infantilized. For some people, this fear of being treated like a baby is worse than the fear of the disease itself.

Proving to your parents that you really *can* do things for yourself, that you really can manage on your own (if that's what you want to do) is one of the hardest things. Independence, perhaps in a specially-adapted flat, might be a better alternative than being treated like a child by your parents in the family home. But it is particularly hard on the parents to have any peace of mind, knowing that their son or daughter is alone in a flat, possibly in real need of help.

Again, there are no easy solutions. Therapy or counselling may be vital to bring fears and deep emotions out into the open.

SEXUAL PROBLEMS IN MEN AND WOMEN

There is no reason why MS should stop or limit your sexual relationship with your partner, or prevent you being a person with sexual desires or needs.

It is true that MS can cause specific sexual problems, but with love, information, communication, an open attitude, patience, and perhaps with the help of new positions or sexual aids, these can be overcome.

It is very important if you are the one with MS that your partner goes on seeing you as a sexually attractive person, and you must do everything to keep yourself that way.

If you think you are unattractive, or doubt your ability to attract or keep a partner, it will have a devastating effect on your self-image or self-esteem. So it is vital to accept and love yourself, so others can feel that way about you too.

Your definition of sexuality may have to be broadened beyond the ability or inability just to have sexual intercourse.

To overcome sex problems you have to communicate openly and honestly with your partner. If you do not share your feelings, your partner may not be aware of your needs. Love and patience on the part of both partners seldom fails to solve problems.

The worst thing you can do is avoid sexual contact. Some couples have a tendency to do this because they are afraid that sex will worsen the condition of the one with MS. On the other hand, they may avoid sex because they do not want it to end in disappointment or frustration, if this has been the outcome of previous encounters.

The danger is that if you become too watchful or worried about what might go wrong, this 'spectatoring' in itself becomes a problem. Performance anxieties always interfere with relaxation and enjoyment, and can inhibit an erection in men and orgasm in women.

Fatigue

This is a major problem for both men and women with MS. However, it is possible to counteract fatigue being a sex problem if you plan your sex life beforehand, even though this does mean that sex will not be spontaneous.

Choose a time of day for sex when your energy is at its highest. It is silly to have sex late at night when you have no energy left. If you make love during the day, rest beforehand. If necessary, get your neighbours to take the children. Avoid interruptions. Try and create a relaxing and erotic atmosphere, it will help make it a more satisfying sexual encounter.

Problems in Men

It is more likely to be men who complain of sexual dysfunction when they have MS than women. This is because any erection disturbance can make the sex act impossible; whereas for women sex is still possible despite any loss of feeling.

It has been estimated that 60 per cent of men with MS do suffer from erection disturbances at some time in the disease, although emotional factors are thought to play a part in about 25 per cent of these cases. About 25 per cent of men with MS do become impotent. Remember that these statistics do not take into account the possibility of stabilizing the disease with the self-help methods described in this book. Like any other MS symptoms, potency can go away and then come back again.

The range of symptoms in men can be anything from minor difficulties in getting and keeping an erection, to disturbances of sensation and ejaculation, to total failure to get an erection.

Ejaculation may be affected because it is also a reflex controlled by the bundle of nerves in the lower spinal cord. Men who have difficulty getting or keeping an erect penis may be less likely to ejaculate.

It is possible for men to be given penile implants, which makes the penis erect all the time and which makes intercourse attainable. There are also certain drugs which give erections which a man can inject into himself.

Men with MS who want to father children may be able to use a technique which involves the artificial stimulation of the penis to ejaculation. The wife is then a candidate for Artificial Insemination by Husband (AIH). Unfortunately, this technique is not available in the UK, but it is in the USA.

Problems in Women

Women with MS may suffer loss of orgasm, diminished libido, or spasticity. They may also have problems with reduced lubrication, anxiety about bladder control, and fatigue. On the other hand, many women with quite severe disability do not experience any of these things, and enjoy normal, satisfying sex.

Intercourse may be more difficult because of spasms of the thighs, and reduced vaginal lubrication. An artificial lubricant, like KY Jelly, usually solves this.

Many women with MS continue to have a normal orgasm reflex. Others, depending on the extent of their neurological damage, may not experience genital orgasm. But it is thought possible for women who do not have a physiological orgasm to nevertheless reach a psychological climax – a sort of 'phantom orgasm' following the partner's excitement and from sharing a common tension release.

There is a definite connection between sexual problems and incontinence. Women tend to be anxious about bladder control when they are having sex. The same bundle of nerves which affects bladder control also controls the orgasm reflex. Women can be afraid of wetting themselves during intercourse, or at orgasm. Or else they feel they have to urinate while in the act of lovemaking. All these things can stop you from letting yourself go.

Overcoming Sexual Problems

Even though sexual intercourse may be hard to achieve, many people find the emotional and psychological pleasure of it vital to a relationship, and it is worth striving to overcome specific difficulties for this reason.

If a man has erection difficulties, intercourse can be achieved by the woman sitting astride her partner and placing his flaccid penis inside her vagina. If she voluntarily contracts her vaginal muscles around his penis, she can hopefully bring about a partial erection.

It may be necessary to try new and different positions to accommodate the partner's specific problems. It should be possible to find a position which is comfortable, and gives pleasure and satisfaction to both partners.

Catheters can be taped against the body so that they are out of the way. A man can wear a condom for hygiene.

If intercourse is too difficult, there are other sexual possibilities to maintain intimacy with your partner. Anything that gives mutual pleasure should be considered right and good, despite some people's attitudes that they might be 'perverted'. These would include oral sex, masturbation, and of course massaging, cuddling, fondling, or any other means of touching and mutual caressing. In a healthy sexual relationship, these would all be additions to sexual intercourse, and not alternatives.

Sexual aids can give pleasure and satisfaction in lovemaking, so you should not treat them with suspicion just because they are manufactured and not 'natural'. Anything that does not actually cause pain in sex, and which gives pleasure to both partners, should be welcomed rather than shunned. After all, no one minds wearing glasses if their eyesight is poor; the same attitude should apply to sexual aids.

If you are embarrassed by the prospect of going into a sex shop, such items can be obtained by mail order. Write to SPOD (see below) for a list of suppliers of sex aids.

Where to Go for Help with Sexual Problems

Counselling and plain information can make a big difference between a miserable sex life and a pleasurable one.

In the UK, there is a group specially set up to help disabled people overcome sexual problems. It is called the Association to Aid the Sexual and Personal Relationships of People With a Disability (SPOD for short).

They have several different leaflets, covering many aspects, including MS. They can be contacted at:

SPOD
286 Camden Road
London, N7 0BJ
Tel: 0171-607 8851

Other Help

A husband, wife, or parent, is probably not the best person to turn to. After all, they are suffering too, with similar feelings of loss, grief and fear. Cry together – but not on their shoulder. It does not always follow that the 'unaffected' partner is the strong one. So it is better to turn to someone outside the immediate situation.

It is important that you do pour your heart out to somebody. The worst thing that you can do is bottle it up inside yourself – that would only add to your anxiety.

It is a good idea to have the safety valve of someone completely removed from your home situation. Someone you have never met before or a faceless voice on the telephone may be the best way for you to open up.

The MS Society Telephone Counselling numbers are:

0171-222 3123 London (24 hours)
0131-226 6573 Scotland
0121-476 4229 Midlands

Julia Segal, a full-time counsellor is at the MS Unit at the Central Middlesex Hospital, London. Tel: 0181-453 2337.

Other bodies concerned with helping in this area are:

British Association for Counselling
1 Regent Place
Rugby CV21 2PJ
Tel: 01788 578328

Carers National Association
20–25 Glasshouse Yard
London EC1A 4JS
Tel: 0171-490 8818

Relate National Marriage Guidance.
For your local Relate, look in your local telephone directory.

Head Office:
Herbert Gray College
Little Church Street
Rugby
Warwicks CV21 3AP
Tel: 01788 73241/60811

Samaritans,
listed in your local telephone directory.

Social Workers

If you do not have a social worker already, contact the Social
Services Department of your local council and they will organize
it. A social worker should be able to help you with practical advice
on aids, adaptation to your home, home helps, etc.

Multiple Sclerosis Society Welfare Officer

If you are a member of the MS Society, they have a welfare officer
who could help you with practical problems. Ask your branch
secretary or write to their head office:

MS Society of Great Britain and Northern Ireland
25 Effie Road
London SW6 1EE
Tel: 0171-610 7171

Psychotherapists

If you find yourself overwhelmed by depression as a result of having MS, your doctor should be able to refer you to a good psychotherapist. In some cases it is possible, though difficult, to get psychotherapy free on the NHS. Even though psychotherapy is very time-consuming and can go on for years, it is worth considering if your personal relationship with your partner or any other problem is giving you distress and you are unable to sort it out on your own.

Finally, it is worth saying again that many people with MS who have followed the various ways of managing the disease have not got worse, and have lived virtually normal personal lives, becoming happy and fulfilled mothers and fathers and able to lead normal family lives.

19

Childbirth and Children

Women with MS thinking of having a baby often worry about having a relapse as a result.

Instead of fearing the worst that having a baby might mean, you could perhaps dream about the best – the sheer joy that a baby brings.

'Joy' is a word that you hear over and over again when women talk about children. I know several women with MS who have had babies since MS was diagnosed. In some, the MS has got worse since having their children. In others, it hasn't. But even those who are quite badly disabled do not regret for one moment that they had children. It would be a greater cause for regret if a woman decided against having children because she has MS.

CAN A WOMAN WITH MS HAVE CHILDREN?

One of the most pressing questions facing a young woman with MS is, 'Can I have children?'

The answer, judging from the many thousands of women with MS who have happily had children, is a definite *yes*.

The 'Baby M' Case

Some doctors in the USA are recommending their female patients with MS not to have a baby in case there is a risk of a relapse as a result.

In the famous 'Baby M' case, a professional woman with only mild MS wanted to pay a surrogate mother to have a baby for her. She gave MS as the reason why she could not have a baby herself.

I have to say that I cannot agree that MS is a good reason not to have a baby yourself. Speaking as a mother, I cannot imagine that a surrogate baby can feel the same to you as one you have carried and delivered yourself.

The 'Baby M' case may have left the idea in the minds of many young women with MS that they cannot have a baby *because* they have MS. This is a tragic idea to give women who would dearly love to have a baby of their own.

This book strongly takes the view that a woman with MS *can* have a baby.

What Risks Are There?

Some doctors say that having a baby when a woman has MS is not so much a medical problem as a social problem. By that, they mean that questions like, 'Who is going to look after the baby?' and 'How much help and support can the husband give?' are more important than the physical side of childbirth, which doesn't in itself cause too many problems.

The risk time for women with MS is not during pregnancy, or even the delivery itself. It is after the baby is born – sometimes many months after, when the broken nights, constant demands of the infant, and tiredness can take their toll. That's why a mother with MS needs more support than normal, from husband, other members of the family, or paid or voluntary help, so the risk of relapse is reduced.

Fertility

If you are healthy enough to have periods, and healthy enough to get pregnant, then the chances are you are healthy enough to have a baby successfully.

Some women with MS lose their periods intermittently, and are unable to get pregnant at those times. But, overall, fertility is not thought to be affected.

If the man has MS, there may be problems in maintaining an erection, or ejaculation, or both. Again, these problems can be intermittent. Many men with MS have fathered children since their MS was diagnosed. (See chapter 18 on sexual problems.)

Pregnancy

Once you have become pregnant, the pregnancy poses no special problems. Many women feel wonderfully well while they are pregnant, once the morning sickness phase has passed.

Some of the symptoms you may get during pregnancy may be perfectly normal and have nothing to do with MS, so don't get unduly worried if, for example, you want to dash to the loo more than usual.

The MS Research Unit at the Central Middlesex Hospital in London has been conducting some informal research about MS and childbirth. They followed 13 pregnant women who passed through the unit. They seemed to have fewer exacerbations of the MS in the second half of the pregnancy than would be expected.

The MS Unit also looked at the available research on the subject and came to the conclusion that pregnancy may actually *delay* relapses. This may possibly be due to a suppressive effect of alpha-fetoprotein, a substance found in the blood of pregnant women.

If someone did have an attack while they were pregnant, they might well think that their MS began or got worse because of the pregnancy. But in fact the figures seem to show that relapses and onset of MS during pregnancy occur no more often than would be expected in young women of childbearing age.

So, it seems safe to say that relapses of MS are not caused by pregnancy.

Ante-Natal Care

There is no reason why you should not follow the same ante-natal care as any other pregnant woman. Some obstetricians put women with MS into the 'high risk' category, and may therefore make you more anxious than need be. The things which make a woman 'high risk' obstetrically have nothing to do with MS (e.g. high blood pressure, diabetes, obesity, etc.).

Your main problem during the ante-natal period will be resisting medically-trained people who will try and persuade you to have a high-tech birth, whether you want to or not.

Decide what kind of birth you want early on in the pregnancy, and make it clear to your hospital ante-natal clinic what you do and don't want.

During the ante-natal period, you might like to join a class of like-minded people, for support and to make new friends who will then have babies the same age as yours.

If you do want a 'high tech' birth, the best thing is to sign on at your hospital ante-natal clinic. If you have leanings towards natural childbirth, you could join an NCT class, or a class at the Active Birth Centre.

The National Childbirth Trust headquarters is at:

Alexandra House
Oldham Terrace
Acton
London W3 6NH
Tel: 0181-992 8637 (enquiry line, Mon–Fri 9.30–4.30)

ParentAbility is a peer support group within the NCT which seeks to empower disabled people as parents and prospective parents. They have a register to enable disabled parents to contact each other, and publish a newsletter. Write to:

ParentAbility
NCT, address as above.

Their centre offers classes for parents-to-be and new parents with their babies. Programme includes pregnancy yoga classes, post natal exercises, and baby massage. They also hire out pools for water birth.

The Active Birth Centre
25 Bickerton Road, London N19 5JT
Tel: 0171-561 9006

Can You Take Vitamins, Minerals and Other Supplements during Pregnancy?

If you have been taking evening primrose oil capsules, plus vitamin and mineral supplements before you got pregnant, it is important not to change anything nutritionally either while you are pregnant or during breastfeeding.

It would be unwise to start taking high doses of vitamins and minerals during the pregnancy unless you continue with these during breastfeeding, as the baby will get used to these high levels and could suffer from a sudden drop if you stopped taking them abruptly.

Supplements of all the B vitamins, plus zinc at 15 mg twice a day would be useful to take during pregnancy.

It is not only perfectly safe to take evening primrose oil during pregnancy, it *may* also be a way of protecting the baby from developing MS later in life. This may sound like an outrageous claim, but there may well be something in it. It is a hypothesis that can neither be proved nor disproved. (See the section below: 'Is there any way of protecting your child against getting MS?')

Drugs During Pregnancy

This book takes the view that drugs which suppress the immune system are positively harmful. The whole book takes a non-drug approach to the management of MS, and this includes pregnancy and childbirth. Any drug can be dangerous during pregnancy, particularly in the first 11 weeks or so.

Drugs which you may have been taking before conception, such as prednisolone, ACTH, or Baclofen, Valium, and Dantrium, should be stopped before trying for a baby. The same applies to drugs used for urinary frequency or incontinence such as Cetiprin or Urispas. Long-term therapies such as azothioprine, cyclosporin and even HBO should all be discontinued before conception.

The Delivery

When you go into labour, the contractions of the uterus are reflex actions, and MS does not affect them. The only problem is that childbirth can be tiring. What kind of delivery you have may depend on the severity of your MS. Unless you are very incapacitated, you have the same choices open to you as any other woman.

If you want a natural childbirth, with no drugs or interference, your biggest problem will probably be finding an obstetrician or a midwife who will agree to you having such a birth.

Unless you are very lucky, most obstetricians and midwives are likely to classify you as 'high risk' or 'complicated'. They are very likely to suggest that you have epidural anaesthesia, or even a planned Caesarean.

These obstetricians who like all their MS women to have Caesareans feel that the uterine muscles of a woman with MS may not be able to push the baby out without help. I do not know of any evidence which says that uterine muscles are affected by MS, or any other kind of paraplegia. A Caesarean is a fairly major operation, involving anaesthetic, and post-operative pain. You are also denied the experience of actually giving birth yourself.

Most hospital births will involve a fair amount of technology. You are likely to be connected to a foetal heart monitor, with bands round your tummy connected to the monitoring machine.

This means you have to lie still during labour, instead of getting into any position you feel like. The foetal heart monitor is to detect whether the baby is getting into distress – but there are other ways of doing this.

The epidural will deaden the pain of the contractions, but it will also deaden feeling anything else from the waist downwards. Someone with MS may find this particularly frightening in case the loss of feeling is MS and not just the anaesthetic.

In a conventional hospital delivery, you would be given a drip whereby a hollow tube is inserted into a vein which gives you a steady supply of dextrose to keep your strength up. Recent research has shown that this can actually *increase* your sensitivity to pain.

It is also quite likely that your delivery will be induced. At the time of the delivery, forceps may well be used, especially if the labour is induced and you have an epidural. Episiotomy – a cut to widen the vaginal opening – often goes with a forceps delivery.

Such a delivery – if you are not having a Caesarean on the operating table – is almost certain to take place on a high delivery bed under bright lights. The medical personnel would all be wearing masks and gowns.

In short, the birth of your baby would be a medical event. The doctors may be offering you these technological aids because they think it will make your birth easier, safer, and less painful. However, there are many women who have been through this kind of birth experience who have felt out of control, as if the baby was being extracted from them.

Natural Birth

If you want your baby's birth to be normal, personal, physiological, and an emotional experience, you will have to be very insistent, and find out which obstetrician will be prepared to take you on for a natural birth.

In a natural childbirth, you trust your body and go along with your instincts. During contractions, you can choose any position you like – on all fours, lying down, lunging forward, being on your side, sitting – anything that feels comfortable. For the delivery itself, you might choose an upright position, such as squatting, hanging squat, or sitting, so that the baby drops down and the descent of the baby is helped by gravity.

When a woman is not interfered with and not disturbed during labour, she is able to secrete the right hormones. These hormones are vital for her feeling of well-being. One of the chemicals she produces is endorphins, which as well as making you feel 'high', also act as painkillers, a bit like morphine.

You do not need strong leg muscles to have a natural birth. You can use a chair or special birthing stool to take your weight. Even if you do squat, it is only for the last couple of contractions anyway. Someone could help you by supporting you under your arms while you do squat.

Of course, there are no drugs whatsoever in a natural birth. The rate of forceps and episiotomy is lower than in high-tech births.

Drugs routinely used in high-tech births do affect the baby, so that they are born more dopey than in a natural birth. Babies born after a natural birth are immediately more alert. This is a good reason in itself to avoid drugs during labour and delivery.

If you want a baby born in this way, ask the NCT or the Active Birth Centre to help you (addresses above).

After the Baby is Born

Immediately after the baby is delivered, it should be given to the mother and they should be together for at least the first hour following birth. Ideally, the father should be there too. This is the optimum time for the 'bonding' to take place which is vital for the relationship between mother and child, and for the healthy development of the baby. Ideally, there should be skin-to-skin contact, so the baby should not be wrapped at this stage. During the first hour, the baby develops the senses of sight, sound, touch, taste and smell, and it instinctively finds the mother's nipple and begins to suck. The risk time for a mother with MS is often much later, when she can become exhausted by looking after a new baby. This is the time you must have support, so you can get enough rest and sleep.

Relapses Around the Time of Birth

There have been several studies concerning the effects of childbirth on the long-term future of women with MS. All of them confirm that there is no difference in long-term disability of women with no baby, with one baby, or with two or more babies.

When there is a relapse in the period surrounding birth, it is more often in the 3-4 months after the birth.

The ARMS figures are that out of 13 pregnant women passing through the MS Research Unit, 7 had a relapse 3-6 months after the birth. Of these, all were back to their previous state within a year. One had a relapse when her child was 12 months old. All of these relapses involved relatively minor symptoms.

The large studies looking at women with MS and childbirth suggest that 40-50 per cent of women have relapses within 3-6 months after the birth. Of these, 80 per cent recover fully, and 20 per cent have some residual damage. This suggests that within a year of the birth nearly all the post-natal relapses have been overcome, and the mother is back to the situation she was in before the pregnancy, as far as the MS is concerned. Remember that these figures do not reflect the possibility of being able to fend off relapses by the self-help methods described in this book.

Breastfeeding

When a woman is breastfeeding she secretes the hormone prolactin. A high secretion of prolactin over a long period of time might be a way to help the immune system recover its previous state. So prolonged breastfeeding may prevent a relapse happening at 3-4 months. It is also very important that the baby gets the mother's colostrum when it is first born. The colostrum is the stuff which precedes actual breast milk, and may play a very important part in building up immunity in the baby.

Prolonged breastfeeding is also the best possible way of protecting the baby. This is the time when myelination is going on. The baby needs specific essential fatty acids for the structure of the myelin to be properly constituted. This period is also the time when the immune system is reaching maturity.

Breastfeeding is pleasurable, and makes the bond between mother and baby even closer and more loving.

If you have any problems with breastfeeding, the best counsellors are from:

La Leche League,
London WC1 3XX
Tel: 0171-404 5011.

Looking After a Baby

People talking about having a baby when you've got MS tend to concentrate on the processes of pregnancy, labour, and the birth itself. But the most physically demanding thing about having a baby is the work involved in looking after it.

Caring for a baby is a 24-hour-a-day job. However you feed your baby, for the first few months you will have very disturbed nights, with only a few hours' sleep at a time. Babies are extremely demanding, and it doesn't get much easier as they grow older.

It is very difficult doing anything else at all with a new baby in the house. All this is very exhausting, even for someone who does not have MS. The joys of a baby are worth it all, but you do need practical help.

Before the baby arrives, make whatever arrangements are necessary to get extra help. It may involve family, friends, neighbours, or paid help.

In addition to human help, try and get your home kitted out with as many labour-saving devices as you can afford – such as a washing machine and drier, dishwasher, microwave oven, etc.

Easing the practical side of having a baby may go a long way to preventing a relapse.

Meeting other new mothers will also help so you have a network of friends and a life outside the home.

If you do have a relapse while your baby is still dependent on you, try and avoid going into hospital as it would be traumatic for the baby to be separated from you. To spare the baby emotional damage, it would be better to stay at home and be nursed there than to leave your baby and be admitted to hospital without him.

To avoid this happening, it is important to try and do everything possible to avoid a relapse. All the therapies in this book have had some success in stabilizing MS and reducing attacks.

WILL THE BABY BE ALL RIGHT?

MS is estimated to be between 5 and 20 times more common among near relatives of someone with MS. MS is not hereditary, but there is a familial link. The fact that MS does run more commonly in families is not special to MS – it happens in many conditions, such as heart disease, hypertension, or cancer.

There is a genetic element in MS. Again, this is the case with many diseases. However, even with those born with the familial predisposition to MS, there is no certainty at all that they will go on to develop the symptoms of MS later on in their lives. There probably has to be a factor X, or many factors, to act on the susceptible person in order for MS to actually manifest itself. There is almost certainly an environmental factor or factors involved.

It is realistic to say that there is an increased risk of a child developing MS later on if the mother has MS. There is less of a chance if the father has MS. But MS is not like haemophilia – it is not inevitably passed from mother to child. The majority of offspring whose mothers or fathers have MS never get the disease.

MY OWN STORY

My son Pascal was born in April 1985. Throughout the pregnancy (as now) I was taking evening primrose oil capsules plus all the vitamins, minerals and trace elements listed in chapters 7 and 8.

I started attending the ante-natal clinic at the local hospital, but opted out when they classified me as 'high-risk' – because I was having my first baby at 38, and had MS. Being classified as 'high-risk' almost certainly meant I would end up having a high-tech birth, which I most definitely did not want. What I wanted was a home birth.

So I continued my ante-natal care with an independent midwife, who came to see me at my home. Even though my partner was Dr Michel Odent, the radical pioneer of natural childbirth, he did not actually deliver our baby as he was not registered as a doctor in Britain at the time.

Pascal was born at home. My labour lasted three hours. I had no medical intervention during the labour or delivery, except that the baby's heartbeats were monitored from time to time with a portable 'Sonicaid'.

For the delivery, I was in the 'hanging squat' position. I was standing up, with my arms around my partner's neck and my hands clasped; then I dropped down into a low squat.

I had no tear, no episiotomy, no post-natal depression. Pascal began sucking at the breast within the first hour. I breastfed on demand, and continued to breastfeed until Pascal was about three and a half, tapering off towards the end. He began mixed feeding on solids at around 7 months.

Even though I was back at work part time from when Pascal was about a year old, and full time from when he was about two, I still continued to breastfeed at night.

I was keen to breastfeed Pascal for as long as possible, as breast milk contains gammalinolenic acid, and I felt this was the best way to build his central nervous system at the crucial age.

Now that Pascal has had this start in life, I'm happy to let him be a normal boy, eating all the kinds of things that children of his age like to eat. After all, I want him to live as normal a life as possible.

As for myself, my ambition is to continue to be a healthy mother to Pascal.

Further Reading

NEWSLETTERS AND MAGAZINES

The best way to keep in touch with what's happening in MS is to read the newsletters and magazines published by the various MS organizations.

MS Matters

This is the lifestyle magazine published six times a year by the MS Society. It includes research updates, feature articles, forum, a letters page, news of the activities of the Society, a penpal section, and many useful advertisements. Available free to members.

Information Leaflets

A wide range of information leaflets covering many aspects of MS is available free from the MS Society's Welfare Department. Write to:

Multiple Sclerosis Society of Great Britain and
   Northern Ireland
25 Effie Road
London SW6 1EE
Tel: 0171-610 7171

Pathways

This is an informative newsletter published by the Multiple Sclerosis Research Centre. Free to members.

The Multiple Sclerosis Resource Centre Ltd
4a Chapel Hill
Stansted
Essex CM24 8AG
Tel: 01279 817101

The Swank MS Foundation Newsletter

Helpful information on how to manage MS in daily life, from the champion of the low-fat diet. Available from:

The Swank MS Foundation
13655 SW Jenkins Road
Beaverton
Oregon 97005
USA

BOOKS

There are many health books which cover in detail topics discussed in this book. These include:

Allergies – Your Hidden Enemy, Theron G Randolph and Ralph W Moss (Thorsons, 1984).

Candida Albicans – Yeast and Your Health, Gill Jacobs (Optima, 1990).

Clinical Ecology, George Lewith and Julian Kenyon (Thorsons, 1985).

Evening Primrose Oil, Judy Graham (Thorsons, 1988).

The Multiple Sclerosis Diet Book, Roy Swank and Barbara Brewer Dugan (Doubleday, USA, 1987).

Multiple Sclerosis, Pregnancy and Parenthood, Judy Graham (Multiple Sclerosis Resource Centre, 1997).

Books on MS

The Complete MS Body Manual, Susie Cornell (1997) available from: PO Box 1270, Chelmsford, Essex CM2 6BQ. £11.90 including p&p).

Multiple Sclerosis – The Natural Way, Richard Thomas (Element, 1995).

Recipes for Health and MS, Geraldine Fitzgerald and Fenella Briscoe (Thorsons, 1996).

Eating and MS – Information and recipes, Susan Fildes (ed) (available from Multiple Sclerosis Resource Centre, 4a Chapel Hill, Stansted, Essex CM24 8AG; tel. 01279 817101).

Emotional Reactions to MS, Julia Segal (available from Multiple Sclerosis Resource Centre; address as above).

Useful Names and Addresses

Multiple Sclerosis Society of Great Britain and Northern Ireland
25 Effie Road
London SW6 1EE
Tel: 0171-610 7171

Wide range of information and advice. Has local branches around the country. Funds major research and welfare. Has respite centres and holiday homes. Membership costs £3 a year.

MS Helpline: 0171-371 8000

The Multiple Sclerosis Society in Scotland
2a North Charlotte Street
Edinburgh EH2 4HR
Tel: 0131-225 3600

The Multiple Sclerosis Society Northern Ireland Office
34 Annadale Avenue
Belfast BT7 3JJ
Tel: 01232 644914

The MS Society Telephone Counselling Lines
(24-hour service via referral from answerphones)
London 0171-222 3123 (24 hours)
Midlands 0121-476 4229
Scotland 0131-226 6573

The Multiple Sclerosis Resource Centre Ltd
4a Chapel Hill
Stansted
Essex CM24 8AG
Tel: 01279 817101

Information, advice, educational material, books and newsletter, *Pathways*. Membership £20 at time of writing.

Multiple Sclerosis (Research) Charitable Trust
Spirella Building
Bridge Road
Letchworth
Herts SG6 4ET
Tel: 01462 484811

Funds research into MS, set up the MS Nurse Forum – specialist MS nurses.

The British Trust for the Myelin Project
4 Cammo Walk
Edinburgh EH4 8AN
Tel: 0131-339 1316

Funds research into demyelinating diseases. Publishes an interesting newsletter.

Federation of MS Therapy Centres

There are around 70 MS therapy centres around the UK. Depending on size, these offer a variety of therapies such as hyperbaric oxygen, diet, counselling, physiotherapy, reflexology, massage, aromatherapy, yoga and continence advice.
    For a full list of all centres in southern England and south Wales:

Bedford MS Therapy Centre
Bradbury House
155 Barkers Lane
Bedford MK41 9RX
Tel: 01234 325781

For centres in the north of England, north and mid-Wales and
southern Ireland:

Northern Association of MS Therapy Centres
c/o G E C Alsthom
PO Box 132
Trafford Park
Manchester M60 1GE
Tel: 0161-872 3422

Scotland has 11 therapy centres. They are listed in the local telephone directories and Yellow Pages under 'MS Therapy Centres'.
Or, for a full list contact:

Association of MS Therapy Centres Scotland
Tayside MS Therapy Centre
Unit 12b
Peddie Street
Dundee DD1 5LB
Tel: 01382 566283

Multiple Sclerosis Healing Trust
PO Box 2469
Shirley
Solihull
West Midlands B90 2QZ
Tel: 0121-422 6162 or 0121-733 8982

Holds clinic in Solihull, where MS people are treated by a doctor
trained in nutritional medicine, offers reflexology, massage, healing, counselling, crystal therapy, magnetotherapy.

The Swank MS Foundation
13655 SW Jenkins Road
Beaverton
Oregon 97005
USA

Useful newsletter

Yoga for Health Foundation
Ickwell Bury
Nr Biggleswade
Bedfordshire SG18 9EF
Tel: 01767 627271

Runs courses for people with MS.

The British Medical Association now recognizes yoga as a 'complementary self-help therapy' and you may be able to get treatment at Ickwell Bury on the NHS. They have a booklet, 'Yoga for People with Multiple Sclerosis', explaining the details.

Also:

The Yoga Therapy Centre
3rd Floor
Royal London Homoeopathic Hospital Trust
60 Great Ormond Street
London WC1N 3HR
Tel: 0171-833 7267

The following clinics use nutritional and environmental medicine to treat MS:

Dr Patrick Kingsley
72 Main Street
Osgathorpe
Leics LE12 9TA
Tel: 01530 223622

The Hale Clinic
7 Park Crescent
London W1N 3HE
Tel: 0171-631 0156

The Castle Street Clinic
36 Castle Street
Guildford
Surrey GU1 3UQ

Biolab Medical Unit
The Stone House
9 Weymouth Street
London W1N 3FF
Tel: 0171-636 5959

The Good Health Clinic
182 Kensington Church Street
London W8 4DP
Tel: 0171-221 2266

The Centre for the Study of Complementary Medicine
51 Bedford Place
Southampton
Hants SO15 2DT
Tel: 01703 334752

and

14 Harley House
Upper Harley Street
London NW1 4PR
Tel: 0171-935 7848

WEBSITES
http://www.mssociety.org.uk

International Federation of Multiple Sclerosis Societies:
http://www.ifmss.org.uk

Jooly's Joint: penpal site run by Julie Howell, who has MS. People
with MS can meet each other via e-mail: ae218@dial.pipex.com

Computer Literate Advocates for Multiple Sclerosis (CLAMS)
Lists all sources of information about MS on the web. Runs the
MS Web Ring. The best route to all info about MS on the internet.
www.clams.org/

MS Crossroads
Essential links and archive data about MS on web worldwide. Run
by Aapo Halko, a Finnish man with MS.
www.helsinki.fi/-ahalko/ms.html

MS Direct
Helps people find their way round information about MS on the
internet. www.aquila.com/dean.sporleder/ms-home/

Colorado HealthNet News
Has Q&A on MS. www.coloradohealthnet.org

The MSers Chat Room
www.geocities.com-klinks.html/msed.html

The 'Red Boa' Society
MS Support Group. www.shore.net/-robertj/boapage.html

MedSupport Friends Supporting Friends (FSF) International
www.medsupport.org/forums.html
24 hour MS Support Hotline. 1-800-793-0766

International Federation of Multiple Sclerosis Societies
Has 36 member societies around the world.
www.infosci.org/MS-internat/FAQ-1.2html

Laurel Highlands Multiple Sclerosis Support Group
For people with MS in south western Pennsylvania.
e-mail: lhmssg@westol.com

The Good Docs List
Lists good doctors state by state.
www.clams.org/goodocs.html

Noreen's Home on the Net
Excellent list of information on MS from the internet compiled by
MS-er Noreen Fogeson.
www.crl.com/-rbarnes/noreen.html

Index